The Dash Diet Cookbook and Complete Beginners Guide

14 Days of Delicious Breakfast, Lunch,
Dinner and Dessert Recipes
[January 2014 Edition]
Patrick Dixon

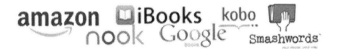

NaturalWay
Publishing

Atlanta, Georgia USA

ISBN 978-1-49493-318-0

9 781494 933180 >

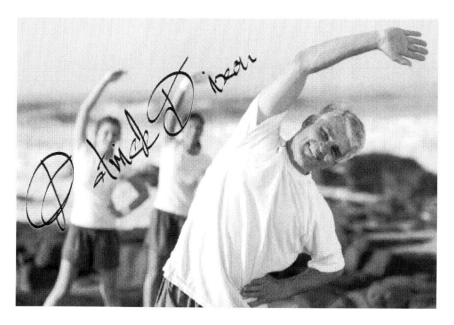

Copyright © 2014 Patrick Dixon

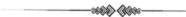

What Our Readers Are Saying

"As far as diets go this is a great one in my book. It helped me lose a lot of weight and regain my confidence."

★★★★☆ Dorothy Adams, LA

"Buying this book was the best thing I did for myself in a long time. This is a guide to a better life."

★★★★☆ Nancy Perez, Minneapolis

"If you want a diet that works then this is the answer to your prayers. I can't thank the author enough for showing me the way to a… weight-less future."

★★★★☆ Sara Mull, San Francisco

Foreword

If you are looking for a diet that can help you in more than one ways then the Dash Diet is the one for you. It helps lower blood pressure, lose weight and manage diabetes, and it also reduces the risk of contracting many other diseases and conditions.

Probably because of the countless diets available out there at the moment, this one is not as popular as it should be quite yet, but as time goes by things are bound to change, since its benefits are so many that more and more people will come to realize its potential.

This book tells you all you need to know about the Dash Diet and explains in detail all its merits. It's divided in four sections. The first section includes general information about metabolic syndrome and the DASH diet, the second focuses on hypertension, the third on weight loss, and the fourth on diabetes. And then come the recipes; lots of recipes. Going on a diet doesn't mean that you should starve yourself, nor does it mean that your food should be taste-free.

Variety is the salt of life, and a healthy life is what everyone is looking for. By reading this guide you'll take a step forward in the right direction.

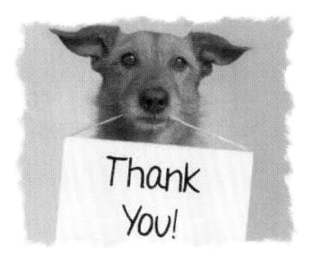

Thank you for downloading my book. Please REVIEW this book. I need your feedback to make the next version better. Thank you so much!

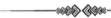

Table of Contents

DISCLAIMER

Introduction

I don't know if it's just me, but the past fifteen years seem to have seen more fad diets than ever before. There have been low-carb diets, high-carb diet, low-fat diets, high-fat diets, fasting diets, juice diets, diets based on how humans used to eat, diets based on how humans should eat. . . it's amazing how many different strategies people have come up with. But even with hundreds of options, thousands of people keep coming back to one single diet because it works. The DASH diet has been around for quite a while, and I'm confident that it will continue to be popular long into the future.

Even though many people think of the DASH diet as a low-sodium one that's generally intended for people with high blood pressure, it has a huge number of benefits and advantages, and almost no drawbacks. It's based on very sound nutritional principles (which is more than many other diets can say), and it's because of this grounding that it's been proven over and over again to be one of the best diets for not only lowering blood pressure, but also losing weight, managing diabetes, and reducing the risk of contracting many other diseases and conditions.

Unfortunately, the DASH diet doesn't get as much credit as it should. Even though it's been voted several times as the best diet by U.S. News and World Report, there are a lot of people who have never heard of it. And there are also a lot of people who think that it doesn't sound as good or effective as many of the fad diets that are out there, simply because the proponents of those fad diets are louder than the thousands of people who have successfully used DASH to help them get back to a healthy weight and blood pressure.

So that's why I'm writing this book—because the DASH diet needs another voice to tell the world how great it is. I hope that after you read this book and discover for yourself just how simple and effective the diet is, you'll become another one of these voices. Read on and decide for yourself if the DASH diet is the best one that's out there—I have confidence that you'll agree this is the case.

And whether you're interested in the DASH diet because you have high blood pressure, are overweight, are dealing with diabetes, all three, or for some other reason, I hope that this book helps guide you to success in becoming healthier!

Sincerely,

Patrick Dixon

How to use this book

This book is divided into four sections. The first section includes general information about metabolic syndrome and the DASH diet, the second focuses on hypertension, the third on weight loss, and the fourth on diabetes. However, no matter which of these conditions you have, I recommend reading through all four sections. I'll be laying out the basics of the DASH diet in the section on hypertension. There'll be more information on the diet in the sections on weight loss and diabetes, but to get a general overview of the diet, you should read the hypertension section as well. And because all of these conditions are related, you'll probably learn a lot in the process!

Finally, after these four sections, I've included a number of recipes to help you get started on the DASH diet. There are recipes for every meal, and I've tried to include a wide variety of different foods so that you get a good idea of what living on the DASH diet is really like. There are a lot of recipe books and websites out there that you can use to supplement these, and I encourage you to give them a try. It's said that variety is the spice of life, and on a diet that doesn't include much salt, you'll need all the spice you can get!

Metabolic syndrome

If I were to ask you what the most prevalent life-threatening condition in America is, what would be your first thought? Heart disease? Lung cancer? AIDS? All of these are good guesses, but there's a very strong argument that it's actually something you might not have heard of: metabolic syndrome. Also dramatically called "syndrome x," metabolic syndrome is actually a combination of several health conditions that you're probably familiar with. Things like obesity, high blood pressure, and high cholesterol.

So what's the deal with these conditions? Why are they all grouped under the umbrella term of metabolic syndrome? Generally, all of these conditions are considered to increase a person's risk of cardiovascular disease, which can lead to things like heart attacks, coronary artery disease, atherosclerosis, and strokes. I hope it's clear why this is something you'd like to avoid!

Because the grouping of these conditions together into metabolic syndrome is a relatively recent thing, different groups still have different definitions of what it is. In general, the following things are taken into account:

- Obesity (often measured by waist size)
- Elevated triglycerides

- Reduced HDL ("good") cholesterol

- Elevated blood pressure

- Elevated fasting glucose

It can also include a measurement of albumin in the blood. The measurements that qualify a person for metabolic syndrome depend on the governing body (the World Health Organization, the American Heart Association, and the International Diabetes Federation all have different guidelines).

One important thing to realize is that most, if not all, of these conditions are closely related. For example, obesity can cause elevated blood pressure. Type II diabetes (related to fasting glucose levels) and elevated triglycerides can be related to poor dietary choices, and obesity is also affected by these choices. While some of these might come about on their own (especially high blood pressure, which can be at least partly genetic or related to non-lifestyle factors), most of them are directly related to things that you can do something about— which means you can significantly reduce your risk of developing cardiovascular disease.

Unfortunately, metabolic syndrome is extremely common in the United States—some people estimate that up to 25% of the population meet the qualifications! That's a huge number of people that are putting themselves at risk. What many of these people don't realize is that there are concrete steps that they can take to not only reduce their risk of cardiovascular disease, but also to take them out of the high-risk population all together.

Understanding cholesterol

While most people know that there's some relationship between high cholesterol and heart disease, many people don't really know much about cholesterol itself and what it means to have high cholesterol. To help you out with this, I'm going to give you a quick primer.

First, it's important to understand that cholesterol itself isn't bad. In fact, it's essential for your body to function. What's bad is when the amounts of cholesterol in your body get out of the ideal range—this is what puts you at risk of cardiovascular disease. Cholesterol itself isn't the culprit; it's having the wrong amount of it.

Second, you need to know that there are two types of cholesterol: HDL and LDL. HDL (high-density lipoproteins) is "good" cholesterol, and actually serves to help prevent heart disease and other potentially debilitating conditions. HDL scours the bloodstream and gets rid of bad cholesterol and helps repair damage to your blood vessels, which can eventually cause arterial disease. LDL (low-density lipoproteins) is "bad" cholesterol, and this is the kind that really causes problems. LDL builds up on the inside of your arteries, causing inflammation and blockage, which can eventually lead to a rupture of your artery, which could form a blood clot that could potentially cause a heart attack.

When you have your cholesterol tested, you usually get four numbers: your HDL levels, your LDL levels, your triglyceride levels, and the total amount of cholesterol. The most important number here is your cholesterol ratio, which you can find by dividing your total cholesterol by your HDL. For example, if your total cholesterol is 250 and your HDL is 50, the ratio is 5:1. The ideal ratio is about 3.5:1, and you should definitely aim to stay under 5:1.

Combining the DASH diet with regular exercise is a great way to manage your cholesterol levels and improve your cholesterol ratio. I won't discuss cholesterol much more in this book, but know that the foods that are included in the DASH diet are heart-healthy and will help you in your battle against high cholesterol.

The basics of a heart-healthy lifestyle

Although there are many consequences of metabolic syndrome, the most significant one is a significantly increased risk of developing cardiovascular disease. Because of this, whether you currently have metabolic syndrome or not, it's a really good idea to lead a heart-healthy lifestyle to reduce your risk of future complications. Things like atherosclerosis, heart attacks, strokes, and coronary artery disease are largely determined by your lifestyle—while they have genetic components, your risk is more strongly affected by the choices that you make in relation to your health.

That's why leading a heart-healthy lifestyle is of the utmost importance. Fortunately, this kind of lifestyle isn't really that hard to maintain! It might seem like a lot of effort at first, but it's actually pretty easy once you get started. A lot of it is related to your diet, which is the factor that will be addressed throughout the rest of this book. Getting exercise is also an important part of a heart-healthy lifestyle, and I'll discuss that a bit, too. But things like quitting smoking, only consuming a moderate amount of alcohol, visiting the doctor for diagnostic checks on a regular basis, taking a daily multivitamin, and managing your stress levels are also important.

This book will help get you started on the path toward a heart-healthy lifestyle. I'll be providing the details of the DASH diet, as well as providing some exercise tips, but the rest is up to you. I highly recommend talking to your doctor about what you can do to decrease your risk of cardiovascular disease. It might not seem like a big deal now, but someday in the future, you might be glad that you did!

What is the DASH diet?

If you're reading this book, it's pretty likely that you already have at least some idea of what the DASH diet is and what it entails. However, in case you're not familiar with it, I'm going to spend the first chapter getting you acquainted with it. Even if you already know something about it, I encourage you to read through this chapter—you never know what you might learn!

First, let's talk about what DASH stands for: the Dietary Approaches to Stop Hypertension. We'll discuss hypertension in the next chapter, but in short, hypertension is chronic high blood pressure. So the DASH diet is a dietary intervention for hypertension. Since becoming popular for hypertension, however, it's also been shown to help with other chronic issues, like weight loss and diabetes, both of which will be discussed in this book.

The history of the DASH diet

Because the DASH diet is so popular, you might expect it to have been around for a long time, but it's actually only been around since the late 90s! In 1992, the National Heart, Lung, and Blood Institute (NHLBI) partnered with five different medical research facilities around the country to conduct a massive, extremely detailed study on the effects of dietary interventions on hypertension.

Over the next five years, extensive data was collected, and, to make a long story short, the group released results showing that the diet plan that they had tested was very effective in reducing the risk and incidence of hypertension. DASH was born! Since then, DASH has undergone additional research, some tweaking, and further development. Offshoots of the original plan now include weight-loss-specific plans and extra-low-sodium plans, which have been shown to further decrease hypertension.

The DASH diet is recommended by the NHLBI, the American Heart Association, the Dietary Guidelines for Americans, and United States guidelines for the treatment of high blood pressure. It's also won the "best diet" award from US News & World Report for the past three years (2011, 2012, and 2013). DASH has received accolades from hundreds of physicians and researchers, and has been successfully used by thousands of dieters. You can't ask for much more support than that!

How does it work?

If you're used to traditional diets, you're probably wondering what the secret is. What's the special ingredient, or the one food that you have to eat every day? Which days do you get to eat a normal diet? How many days do you have to spend on a juice fast? Well, you'll be happy to know that the DASH diet is different—there's no trick, no catch, no special foods. It's just a balanced diet that's low in sodium, low to moderate in fat content, and high in healthy carbohydrates and lean sources of protein. That's it—it's really that simple. You don't even have to count calories!

More specific guidelines will be presented later in the book, and I'll help you tailor the plan to fit your specific needs.

Is it safe?

This is always an important consideration when you're thinking about starting a diet. Some diets are effective, but come with some pretty serious health risks. Others might not be suitable for people with certain conditions. However, because the DASH diet is balanced and doesn't require cutting foods out of your diet, it's generally considered to be very safe.

Of course, before you start any diet, you should talk to your doctor to make sure that you're healthy enough to do it. Talk to them about your current health, your medications, and your exercise habits (if you're not exercising much now, it's an especially good idea to get a physical exam to make sure that you're healthy enough to undertake some exercise).

I'll also mention here that transitioning to a high-fiber diet like this one can make some people uncomfortable; if you're not used to this kind of food, you might experience bloating or gas, diarrhea, constipation, or other digestive difficulties. Be patient, and don't worry—these will pass, and you'll be well on your way to meeting your health goals with the DASH program.

What is hypertension?

I mentioned in the last section that hypertension is another word for chronic high blood pressure. But exactly what that means requires some explanation. This chapter will help you understand what hypertension is, learn how to figure out if you have it, and what that might mean for you.

Blood pressure: an introduction

So what, exactly, is blood pressure? This is something that a lot of people don't actually understand very well. Blood pressure is a measurement of the pressure that circulates blood exerts on the walls of your blood vessels. Generally, arterial pressure is what's measured by your doctor (there's a major artery that runs down the inside of your arm, which is why blood pressure is usually measured there).

Blood pressure is one of the vital signs, and it's important because it affects your body's circulation, which is what keeps oxygen and nutrients flowing to all of your organs, including your heart and your brain. Many conditions have been linked to chronic high blood pressure, including stroke, heart attacks, kidney failure, and even eye problems. Persistently low blood pressure can also cause problems, including dizziness and fainting.

Because of all the risks that abnormal blood pressure poses, it's very important to keep your blood pressure under control. Unfortunately, there are a lot of things in our culture that tend to increase blood pressure, including poor diet, stress, obesity, some medications, and hormonal issues.

Understanding blood pressure values

If you've had your blood pressure taken by a physician, you were given two values, like "140 over 95" or "133/98." If you've never learned what these numbers mean, this might not help you very much. So I'll break it down for you.

The first number in the blood pressure reading is your systolic pressure, which represents the maximum amount of pressure in your blood vessels at the point where the measurement was taken (usually the brachial artery, on the inside of the upper arm). The second number in the reading is your diastolic pressure, which represents the low end of the pressure changes in the artery. Why does your blood pressure change like this? It has to do with the pumping action of the heart, which moves blood throughout your entire body. The blood pressure changes in different parts of your body cause your blood to flow. Blood pressure measurements are taken in mmHG, or "millimeters of mercury," which is a standard unit of pressure.

Now that you have a better idea of what these numbers mean, we can talk about *your* values. According to the Mayo Clinic, there are four levels of blood pressure values. You can see these values in the table below.

Category	Systolic pressure (mmHG)	Diastolic pressure (mmHG)
Normal	90–119	60–79
Prehypertension	120–139	80–89
Stage I hypertension	140–159	90–99
Stage II hypertension	160+	100+

It's important to note that you don't have to have a systolic *and* diastolic in one of the ranges for quality for that category; you only need one. For example, if you get a reading of 121 over 78, you're in the prehypertension category.

Obviously, it's best to be in the normal range. Even if you're in the prehypertension range, you're at increased risk of various conditions, including heart disease and stroke. And if you're in stage II hypertension, you're at serious risk. If your systolic pressure is above 160 mmHg, you need to undergo some serious blood-pressuring-lowering interventions as soon as possible.

What causes hypertension?

There are a lot of different things that can cause your blood pressure to rise into the danger zone. Obviously, diet plays an important role—a diet high in salt, saturated fat, trans fat, and other unhealthy substances can significantly increase your risk of developing hypertension. But there are also other things that can contribute, too, including genetics, long-term exposure to stress, and being overweight.

But just because you experience these things doesn't mean that you'll develop high blood pressure right away. There's an interview with a woman named Izzy on WebMD, and she discusses how her blood pressure was normal for the first 10 years of being overweight! It wasn't until a decade later that she started to see elevated blood pressure readings, which prompted her to start dieting. She went from 130 / 80 down to 105 / 55 in just two years with the DASH diet. No matter what the cause of your hypertension is, the DASH diet will help you get it under control.

The DASH diet for hypertension

The DASH diet was originally created to help people with chronically high blood pressure to get it under control and reduce the health risks associated with hypertension, and this is what the diet is most widely known for. Using the DASH diet will help you get your hypertension under control, and it can also serve as a preventative measure if you're in the pre-hypertensive stage.

The specifics of the diet

Now that you have a better understanding of what hypertension is, it's time to get into the diet itself. As I mentioned before, this is quite a simple diet; it's full of fresh fruits and vegetables, whole grains, and lean sources of protein. The anti-hypertension variant of the diet also restricts the amount of sodium that you eat—and if you consume a lot of salt right now, the amount might seem frighteningly low. But you'll get used to it! And once you've adjusted to the new mainstays of your diet, you'll realize that they taste great, even without salt.

One of the most appealing parts of the DASH diet is that it doesn't require any calorie counting. Instead, it's based on the number of servings of each category of food that you should eat every day. This makes it easy to follow, flexible, and very versatile.

The DASH diet uses the following table to determine your proper intake each day.

Food	Servings on 2000-calorie diet	Servings on 1600–3100 calorie diet
Low-fat or non-fat dairy	2–3	2–4
Vegetables	4–5	4–6
Grains and grain products	7–8	6–12
Leans meats, fish, and poultry	2 or less	1.5–2.5
Fruits	4–5	4–6
Nuts, seeds, and legumes	4–5 / week	3–6 / week
Fats and sweets	limited	2–4

As you can see, this is a very simple diet. You'll notice that there are two different columns, both with a range of possible servings. This is because many different people are on the DASH diet, and everyone has different calorie requirements. Some people can lose weight and reduce their blood pressure on 3100 calories per day. Others need to go down to 1600. Most people, however, will be around 2000 calories per day. (If you need to determine how many calories you should be eating for weight loss, consult the next section.)

If you're wondering what a serving is, you can check out the following list, which has been adapted from *The DASH Diet Action Plan* by Marla Heller, one of the most popular books on the DASH diet.

- Carbohydrates
    - 1 slice of bread
    - 1/3 cup cooked pasta, or rice
    - 1/2 cup cooked cereal, corn, or potatoes
    - 1/4 bagel
    - 1 oz. dry cereal
    - 1/2 English muffin
    - 2 cups popcorn
- Fruit
    - 4 oz. fruit juice
    - 1 small piece of fruit (like a small apple or orange)
    - 1/4 cup dried fruit
    - 1/2 up canned fruit

- 1 cup diced raw fruit
- Vegetables
    - 1/2 cup cooked vegetables
    - 1 cup leafy greens
    - 6 oz. vegetable juice
- Low-fat or non-fat dairy
    - 8 oz. milk
    - 1 oz. reduced-fat cheese
    - 1/2 cup cottage cheese
- Beans, nuts, and legumes
    - 1/4 cup beans, nuts, or seeds
    - 2 Tbsp. peanut butter
- Lean meat, fish, or poultry
    - 1 oz. of meat / fish / poultry
    - 1 egg
    - 2 egg whites
- Fats and sweets
    - 1 Tbsp. salad dressing
    - 1 Tbsp. butter or oil
    - 2 small cookies

While this doesn't cover everything that you might eat in a day, it should give you enough of an idea to convert anything to the serving scale used by the diet.

A sample DASH diet plan

The guidelines listed above should make it pretty easy to come up with your own DASH diet plan. But just to give you an example, I'll give you a sample diet for a day. This diet is based on the 2000-calorie intake, and includes a wide variety of different foods.

- Breakfast: 1/2 cup of cooked oatmeal with 8 oz. low-fat milk, a handful of raspberries, and 6 oz. vegetable juice.

- Morning snack: One apple with 2 Tbsp. peanut butter, 1/2 cup cottage cheese, and one piece of whole-wheat toast.

- Lunch: 2/3 cup cooked whole-wheat pasta with 1 cup cooked vegetables (like onions, peppers, and zucchini) and 1 Tbsp. olive oil.

- Afternoon snack: 2 cups popcorn, 8 oz. fruit juice, and 1 oz. low-fat cheese.

- Dinner: 1/3 cup rice, 2 oz. grilled salmon, 1 cup salad, and 1 Tbsp. low-fat salad dressing.

- Evening snack: 1/2 English muffin and 1/4 cup dried fruit.

As you can see, this doesn't look like a normal diet plan. You actually get to eat a reasonable amount of food! One of the reasons for this is that the standard DASH diet doesn't focus on losing weight—it focuses on lowering your blood pressure. If you're interesting in losing weight, however, you'll need to restrict your calorie intake a bit (see the next chapter for more information using the DASH diet to lose weight).

Another important thing to notice is that there are a lot of servings of carbohydrates in this diet. For the 2000-calorie diet, 7–8 servings of carbohydrates are recommended. With the recent proliferation of low-carbohydrate diets, this might not seem like a good idea, but something that a lot of people don't tell you about these low-carb diets is that, although they work very quickly, they aren't very good for you. If you don't undertake a low-carbohydrate diet with a very scientific understanding of what you're doing, you're likely to have quite a few health problems that result. So don't immediately think "this diet has *way* too many carbohydrates to be effective!" The low-carb craze is a fad, while eating a balanced diet and exercising a lot are never going to go out of style. They'll always work as weight-loss and health-management strategies.

One of the best parts of the DASH diet is that it's so flexible—if you don't like cottage cheese, you can have yogurt instead. If you're not a fan of salmon, have a lean cut of pork. Can't stand vegetable juice? Have a few baby carrots. Because there are no foods that are absolutely required on the diet plan, you can customize it to suit your needs very easily.

Determining your sodium intake

You may notice that sodium levels, which I mentioned earlier are very important, are not presented in the table. Again, this is because people are used for different levels of sodium consumption, and people adjust on different schedules. In 2009, the Centers for Disease Control and Prevention estimated that the average American consumes 3,436 mg of salt every day. That's a lot! The goal for anyone on the DASH diet for hypertension is to get down to 1500mg per day, which is a pretty low number to aim for.

The CDC recommends that all adults aim for around 1500mg of sodium intake per day. That's pretty low if you usually have 4000mg or more! That's why it's a good idea to take steps down. If you regularly eat a huge amount of salt, you should aim to limit yourself to 3000mg per day. After a while, that will become easier, and you should aim for 2300mg. Finally, you can step all the way down to 1500mg per day, your final goal. How long you spend at each step depends on how comfortable you are with reducing your sodium intake, but I'd recommend no more than two weeks. And if you're already in stage I hypertension, a shorter amount of time, like a week, is probably better.

The only way to know how much sodium you're consuming, both before and during the diet, is to check food labels and record the amount of sodium that's in everything that you eat. Doing this for a few days before you start the diet will give you a good baseline measurement of how much salt you eat in a day. Then, once you start the diet, you can keep track every day (or, to make it easier, three to four days a week) to make sure that you're sticking to your goal.

There are plenty of apps that you can download on your phone that will help you keep track of things like this (personally, I like Lose It!), but you can also just use a small notebook that you keep with you all day. No matter how you decide to do it, tracking your sodium intake is crucial for lowering your blood pressure with the DASH diet.

The importance of exercise

You'll notice that I talk about exercise quite a bit in this book—that's because exercise is such an important facet of any diet, no matter the goal. If you're trying to control your blood pressure, exercise is a key component of your strategy—improving your cardiovascular fitness is not only likely to reduce your blood pressure, but it also reduces your risk of heart disease from other sources, as well.

If you've been classified as suffering from hypertension, it's important to talk to a doctor before starting an exercise plan. This is to make sure that your health is good enough for you to start exercising and to bring any potential risk factors to the attention of your doctor.

When it comes to lowering your blood pressure and other cardiovascular health issues, the value of exercise cannot be overstated. Exercise is important for general health, too, but if your heart and blood vessels are at risk from high blood pressure, it's an especially good idea to strengthen them through exercise.

So what kinds of exercises are good for strengthening your cardiovascular system? In general, you're going to want to engage in aerobic exercises. These are things like jogging, cycling, swimming, rowing, and other activities that keep your heart rate elevated for an extended period of time. How you decide to get your exercise is up to you—maybe you want to use an elliptical or a stair-climber at a gym. Maybe you want to start running or swimming laps. Even walking is good for your heart! Exercise doesn't have to be exhausting and painful for it to be beneficial. In fact, if you're in stage 1 or 2 of hypertension, it's a good idea to keep your exercise intensity quite low (and to talk to your doctor before you start).

If you currently don't exercise very much, you might just start with a small amount of exercise at a time—go for a brisk 15-minute walk or ride a stationary bike for 20 minutes. You can even just start with 10 minutes of exercise at a time. When you're beginning an exercise program, it's also a good idea to take some time between your workout sessions to let your body rest. As you gain fitness, however (and you will!), you can start exercising longer and more often. You don't have to start training for a marathon, but engaging in a 60-minute bout of exercise is a great way to gain a lot of benefits for your cardiovascular system.

The CDC recommends 2 hours and 30 minutes of moderate-intensity exercise per week for adult. To get to this benchmark, all you have to do is exercise for 30 minutes five times a week. That might sound like a lot, but if you work up to it, it'll be totally reasonable! You can even break it up into 10-minute segments if it makes it easier for you. If you decide that you'd like to try some higher-intensity exercise, you can meet the CDC recommendations with only 1 hour and 15 minutes of exercise a week. So if you're running, swimming laps, or playing an active sport, you're really doing yourself a favor!

Finally, the CDC lists a range of exercise values for even greater health benefits—to meet these recommendations, you'll need to engage in moderate-intensity exercise for five hours or a week, or vigorous exercise for 2 hours and 30 minutes. I know this seems like a lot, but we're talking about your health here—it's important!

Monitoring your blood pressure

If you have high blood pressure—or you're at increased risk of it—you should have your blood pressure checked on a regular basis. Exactly how regular should be discussed with your doctor, but if you've ever had a blood pressure reading on the high side of normal, you should try to have it checked every year by a professional. If you've never had a high reading, once every three or four years should suffice. However, as you get older, you're at increased risk of developing high blood pressure, so once you reach the age of 40, it's a good idea to get it checked more often; every two years should be good.

There are many home blood pressure monitoring systems on the market that you can use to keep track of your blood pressure without going to see your physician. You can always buy a simple sphygmomanometer (the blood pressure cuff your doctor uses) and learn how to use it—if you learn how to do it correctly, you can be assured of accurate readings (it might seem complicated, but it's actually pretty easy to use the sphygmomanometer). There are also automatic blood-pressure monitors that require no action on your part other than pushing a button. There's quite a bit of debate over whether these are accurate, so it's a good idea to make sure that you're getting a high-quality one that's FDA-approved, and follow the instructions provided by the manufacturer.

A manual sphygmomanometer will probably cost between $20 and $30, but an automatic machine could run you up to $100, though you can find several models that are closer to $50. And of course, you can always just go see your doctor to get a full health check-up, which is probably a good idea anyway. Something that's increasingly common is blood pressure screenings at pharmacies and other public places—if you ever have the chance to get a free screening, take it!

The DASH diet for weight loss

Even though this diet was originally developed to help people get their high blood pressure under control, it's been shown over and over to be a very effective weight loss tool as well. All kinds of people have used it to manage their weight, from teen girls to grown men, and there are some pretty amazing success stories. One woman documented her weight loss process with the DASH diet on YouTube, and it's absolutely amazing to see her go from weighing 230 pounds to being just under 145 with normal blood pressure! The transformation is astounding, and has inspired a great many people to use the DASH diet as a central component of their weight loss process. Whether you're looking to lose 9 pounds or 90, this is a diet that will help you meet your goals without resorting to some of the unhealthy or extremely inconvenient strategies that other diets use.

How do I know if I'm overweight?

This is something a lot of people don't know, so I'll address it here, before going onto the mechanics of weight loss and the diet itself. There are a few different ways to determine if you're overweight, but the simplest one is to use your body mass index, or BMI. BMI is essentially a way to estimate the proportion of your body that's made up of lean tissue versus the amount that's made up of fat. That sounds complicated, but it's actually quite simple; all you have to do is enter your height and weight into the following formula:

$$BMI = (\text{weight in lbs.} / (\text{height in in.}^2)) \times 703$$

You can also use one of the many calculators online, such as the one at http://www.mayoclinic.com/health/bmi-calculator/NU00597. Once you've figured out your BMI, the rest of the process is simple. If your BMI is between 18.5 and 24.9, you're in the healthy range. If you're at 25 or over, though, you're in the overweight category. And if you score 30 or more, you're classified as obese. I've seen a few charts list values of 40 or over as extremely or morbidly obese, but that's less common.

But don't worry! Even if your BMI is higher than it should be, you can lose weight and get back down below 25. It might seem like a BMI of 25 is impossibly far away, but you can do it—it just takes commitment and some patience.

How weight loss works

Something that many people don't understand is why weight gain occurs, and how it can be reversed and prevented. One of the reasons for this is that many fad diets don't address the most important cause of weight gain! Using the DASH diet, however, will allow you to lose weight in a healthy, stable manner that's based on thousands of hours of research and millions of pounds lost.

So, let's go over the basics. Why do people gain weight? In short, because they consume more calories than they burn. We get calories from the food that we eat, and we burn those calories for energy—the beating of your heart takes energy, as does your breathing; so does walking, jogging, lifting weights, swimming, and every other form of exercise.

If you're eating more calories than you're burning in a day, you're creating what's called a calorie surplus, and your body is storing those extra calories so it can use them later. The problem is that you don't always use them later! If you consume more calories than you burn, even if just by a little bit, your weight will slowly creep up over time until you've made it to the "overweight" category before you know it. (If you're wondering why our body stores calories that we don't use, most people think that it's an evolutionary adaptation for when food was more scarce during the winter.)

What's the solution to this? Burning more calories than you consume! By doing this, your body will need to use the calories that it's stored up for energy, and you'll create a calorie deficit—which, over time, results in weight loss. It's that simple. Let's take a look at how to plan your own weight loss diet.

Determining how many calories you should be consuming

Obviously, figuring out how many calories you should be consuming in a day is of the utmost importance when it comes to creating a calorie deficit. If you don't know how many calories you're burning in a day, it's really hard to know how much you should be consuming. Fortunately, there are some simple tools that will help you figure it out. Just plug your weight, height, and age into this equation:

- Women: 655 + (4.35 x weight in lbs.) + (4.7 x height in in.) - (4.7 x age in years)
- Men: 66 + (6.23 x weight in lbs.) + (12.7 x height in in.) - (6.8 x age in years)

This will give you your basal metabolic rate, or BMR, which estimates the number of calories that you burn at rest on any given day. This means that you'd burn this many calories if you were to sleep all day–it's the number of calories you need just to stay alive and functioning. Now, we need to figure out how many calories you burn from exercise. For this, just multiply your BMR by a value that corresponds to your activity level.

- Sedentary (little or no exercise): BMR x 1.2
- Lightly active (light exercise 1–3 days / week): BMR x 1.375
- Moderately active (moderate exercise 3–5 days / week): BMR x 1.55

- Very active (hard exercise 6–7 days / week): BMR x 1.725
- Extra active (very hard exercise or physical job): BMR x 1.9

Once you've multiplied your BMR by the associated value, you have an estimate of the number of calories that you burn every day. Pretty simple, huh?[1]

Okay, now that we've figured out how many calories you burn every day, we can find out how many you need to consume to lose weight. A healthy rate of weight loss is one pound a week—that might seem slow, but it's much easier to maintain than going faster, and it's less likely to cause any health issues, so it's definitely the rate that I (and most health professionals) recommend. In order to lose one pound per week, you need to create a deficit of 500 calories each day. So just subtract 500 from the number you calculated above, and you have your daily calorie goal. That's all there is to it!

To sum it all up, here are the three steps you need to figure out how many calories you should be consuming to lose one pound per week:

1. Determine your basal metabolic rate using the equation above.
2. Multiply your BMR by a factor based on how active you are.
3. Subtract 500.

---

[1]I'll note here that you can also get a much more accurate measurement of your BMR from a professional. There are a number of professionals, including personal trainers and physicians, that can do this for you.

Using the DASH diet to lose weight

You might be asking yourself why I'm writing so much about calories when I said earlier that one of the best parts of the DASH diet is that you don't have to count calories. There are DASH plans for several different levels of caloric intake, which allow you to choose the plan that most closely approximates the number of calories that you need per day.

So let's say your BMR is 1900, and you don't exercise, so you multiply it by 1.2. After subtracting 500, you get a daily calorie goal of 1780. In the table below, I give serving guidelines for 1200-, 1400-, 1600-, 1800-, 2000-, 2600-, and 3100-calorie diets. 1800 is a bit too high, but it's pretty close to 1780. What I recommend is using the 1800 plan, but subtracting a serving or two of lean meats, high-fiber carbohydrate, or low-fat dairy. That will bring you closer to your goal of 1780, and you'll be on your way to weight loss! No matter how many calories you should be consuming in a day, this table will help you figure out how many servings of each food group you should be consuming. This table was adapted from one developed by the National Heart, Blood, and Lung Institute (a part of the National Institutes of Health), so the food groups are slightly different than the ones that I outlined above. They're similar enough that you shouldn't have any problems converting, though.

Food Group	1,200 calories	1,400 calories	1,600 calories	1,800 calories	2,000 calories	2,600 calories	3,100 calories
Grains	4–5	5–6	6	6	6–8	10–11	12–13
Vegetables	3–4	3–4	3–4	4–5	4–5	5–6	6
Fruits	3–4	4	4	4–5	4–5	5–6	6
Low-fat dairy	2–3	2–3	2–3	2–3	2–3	3	3–4
Lean meats	3 or less	3–4 or less	3–4 or less	6 or less	6 or less	6 or less	6–9
Nuts, seeds, and legumes	3 per week	3 per week	3–4 per week	4 per week	4–5 per week	1	1
Fats and oils	1	1	2	2–3	2–3	3	4
Sweets	3 or less per week	3 or less per week	3 or less per week	5 or less per week	5 or less per week	2 or less	2 or less

Changes to the standard diet for weight loss

Although the DASH diet for weight loss is very similar to the diet for controlling blood pressure, there are a couple of small changes that I recommend if weight loss is your primary goal. These are minor changes, so you'll still be getting the blood pressure benefits, but they might help you just a little bit more if you're trying to lose weight.

First, replace one serving of carbohydrates every day with an extra serving of lean meat. Increasing your protein intake when you're trying to lose weight is advantageous, as processing protein-rich foods actually require a few more calories than processing carbohydrates. This doesn't make a huge difference, but over the course of months or years, it can add up to quite a bit. Increased protein will also help you with building muscle, which is crucial (as is discussed in the next section).

Second, you may want to adjust your dietary practices based on your exercise. Because exercise is such an integral part of weight loss, it's likely to play a pretty large role in your diet strategy—and because of this, your metabolism will probably start to change a bit. When you start exercising more often, you will build muscle and change your body composition—you will also start to burn more calories throughout the day to help your body cope with the activity. To make sure that your diet is still supporting your needs, you may need to increase your caloric intake a bit if you feel hungry or tired all day. This is totally normal. Another thing that might help is to eat right after workouts—having protein is a really good idea, as it will help your body recover from the exercise and prepare you for the next session.

Don't be afraid to experiment—everyone's body is different, and if you think you might know how to better support your weight loss with your diet, go for it!

Exercise and weight loss

In the previous chapter, I discussed how exercise is really important for lowering your blood pressure. As true as that is, it's even *more* important for weight loss. So many people start losing weight with a diet, but then find their motivation and discipline waning, causing them to start gaining again. If most of these people had included a solid amount of exercise in their weight loss plan, they would've been less likely to experience this problem. One of the best parts about exercise is that after you make it past the first difficult part, you start to really enjoy it! Exercise brings with it a lot of physical health benefits, but it's also a stress reliever and can give you a bit of a high after a good workout. It's an indispensable part of safe, effective, and long-lasting weight loss.

How much you exercise depends a lot on your weight loss plan, schedule, and physical health. As I mentioned in the last chapter, it's very important to talk to a doctor before starting an exercise plan to make sure that you're not putting yourself at risk. Once you've gotten the okay, though, it's time to get started!

As I said earlier, it's good to increase your exercise gradually, especially if you have high blood pressure, are significantly overweight, or have any other health conditions that could complicate your exercise. For the most part, the recommendations that I outlined in the previous chapter apply here, too. Starting with walking for even

15 minutes at a time is a really great way to gear your body up for exercise (walking is actually a great weight-loss exercise). Just follow the instructions for ramping up your exercise gradually.

However, if you're aiming to lose weight, your exercise goals will be different than if you're just trying to lower your blood pressure. You should be aiming to get up to the second level of the CDC recommendations (5 hours per week of moderate-intensity exercise or 2 hours 30 minutes of vigorous exercise) to make sure you're burning enough calories. Another important way in which the exercise plans differ is that for weight loss, you should also be doing muscle-building exercise twice a week.

Building up muscle isn't just an aesthetic thing—it actually plays a pretty important role in your weight loss. While you're at rest, muscle burns more calories than fat, which means that if you replace a pound of fat with a pound of muscle, you'll be burning more calories throughout the day. It'll also allow you to complete more activity throughout your day, helping burn even more calories. And, of course, there is also a wealth of other benefits to building muscle—you'll be able to continue doing your daily activities longer into your life, and you'll be less likely to sustain an injury when you're doing something strenuous.

The most obvious example of muscle-building exercise is weight lifting. But if you're not interested in hitting the gym, you have some other options, too—you can take an intense yoga class (something like the Vinyasa or Ashtanga varieties), or do some heavy yard work (if it involves digging, shoveling, or moving heavy things). You can also do some body-weight exercises, like push-ups, squats, and sit-ups. No matter what you decide to do, aim to complete this kind of exercise twice a week. You might be really sore after the first few times, but stick with it! As you get stronger, it'll become easier.

A sample DASH diet plan

As I did in the last chapter, I'll provide you with a sample DASH diet plan for a day that will show you what kind of foods you can expect to be eating if you're trying to lose weight with the DASH diet. Again, this is for a goal of around 2,000 calories per day.

- Breakfast: 1 egg, 1 piece of whole-wheat toast, 1 oz. cheese, and 8 oz. fruit juice.

- Morning snack: 1 cup baby carrots, 1/2 bagel, and 1/4 cup dried fruit.

- Lunch: 2/3 cup rice, 1 cup cooked vegetables, and 1 Tbsp. olive oil.

- Afternoon snack: 1 small orange, 1/2 cup cottage cheese, and 1/4 cup mixed nuts.

- Dinner: 2 oz. lean meat, 1 cup salad with handful of strawberries, and 1 Tbsp. low-fat salad dressing.

- Evening snack: 1 cup diced mixed fruit, 1 oz. dry cereal, and 8 oz. milk

This is quite similar to the diet plan that you saw previously, but you'll notice that there's an extra serving of lean protein in the egg for breakfast, and one less serving of carbohydrates.

The DASH diet for diabetes

The American Diabetes Association estimates that almost 26 million people in the United States have diabetes—that's over 8% of the entire population! And even more worrying, they estimate that 79 million people have prediabetes, meaning that they don't have diabetes yet, but that they're at risk of developing it in the future. That's over a hundred million people that could be dealing with diabetes in the foreseeable future.

Even if you don't have diabetes, it's important for you to keep in mind that you might be at risk for developing it in the future. There are a lot of risk factors that can increase your chances, including being over the age of 40, being overweight, and high blood pressure. As you can see, this list is similar to the list of symptoms of metabolic syndrome—again, I hope that you see how closely all of these issues are connected.

Understanding diabetes

Unfortunately, diabetes is often misunderstood. There are two main kinds of diabetes, and a lot of people don't totally understand the difference between the two—however, this is an important distinction, so I'm going to set the record straight.

First, you need to understand what insulin is. Insulin is a hormone—a chemical messenger that your body uses to send messages. Insulin sends specific messages about your blood sugar—when insulin rises, your body stores more carbohydrates, decreasing your blood sugar. Once your blood sugar levels have fallen, insulin stops being released by the body, making sure that these levels don't fall too low. If insulin isn't correctly doing its job, your blood sugar can rise to dangerous levels; and if it stays there, you can suffer some pretty unpleasant consequences, including cardiac arrhythmias, a feeling of mental sluggishness, and even coma. The effects aren't always this drastic, but over an extended period of time, it can be very bad.

Type 2 diabetes is the kind that most people are talking about when they discuss diabetes. It's a condition that's contracted—you're not born with it. The risk factors that I listed above are the risk factors for this kind of diabetes. In type 2 diabetes, one of two problems is present. First, you might not produce enough insulin. Second, your cells might not respond very well to insulin (this is called insulin resistance). Either of these conditions can cause blood sugar to increase. Your diet can contribute to these conditions if it contains a lot of carbohydrates that are high on the glycemic index— things like refined white sugar, high-fructose corn syrup, white bread, white potatoes, and regular pasta. These causes large fluctuations in your blood sugar, which causes havoc with your insulin cycle.

Type 1 diabetes is a bit different—it often shows up early in a person's life, such as in their teens. In this type of diabetes, the body loses the ability to produce insulin. This is a lifelong condition, and needs to be treated with daily insulin injections to provide the body with the necessary hormones to manage blood sugar. Because this is something that you're born with and requires a very specific medical treatment, I won't be talking about type 1 any further.

In contrast, you have a lot of control over type 2 diabetes, especially when it comes to reducing your risk of developing it. Most of the risk factors for type 2 are related, at least in part, to your diet, which means that eating a healthy, balanced diet like the DASH diet will go a long way toward preventing diabetes, meaning that you won't have to deal with insulin injections, finger sticks, and potential complications.

Diagnosing diabetes

To find out if you have diabetes, you'll have to have a blood test done by your doctor. However, there are a few symptoms that you can watch for to see if you should get yourself checked out. Here are some of the warning signs:

- frequent urination;
- increased thirst;
- constant fatigue;
- unexplained weight loss;
- slow healing of cuts;
- blurred vision.

If you have more than a couple of these symptoms, or you start experiencing them suddenly, you might want to make an appointment to speak with your doctor about getting tested for diabetes. Leaving this condition undiagnosed can be quite dangerous, as you'll find out later on in the next section.

Managing type 2 diabetes

To keep type 2 diabetes under control, it's best to keep your blood sugar levels as consistent as possible—big rises and dips are what often causes problems for diabetics. So diabetics need to closely monitor their blood sugar levels to make sure that they don't get into the danger zones. Beyond this, the methods for managing the condition generally fall into two categories: lifestyle changes and medications.

Lifestyle changes include things like regular exercise, which helps lower blood sugar, and a balanced diet that helps keep blood sugar level. Certain types of foods help keep your blood sugar from swinging up or down quickly, and including a lot of these foods in your diet will help you keep your diabetes under control. Fortunately, there are a lot of these foods on the DASH diet plan!

Medications have various effects, but most either stimulate your pancreas to produce more insulin or increase your cells' sensitivity to the hormone. There are a lot of different diabetes medications, and if you think you might need one, I encourage you to talk to your doctor, because even a short review of them is beyond the scope of this book.

Another important part of managing type 2 diabetes is regular blood sugar monitoring. There are a few different ways to measure your blood sugar, but a simple finger stick is the most common way. Again, this is something that you should talk to your doctor about.

A personal friend of mine was once sent to the hospital from a music festival because of her diabetes. Her condition had been well controlled for many years, but being in a new situation and not eating normally caused her blood sugar to go way out of the safe zone. I share this story only to impress upon you the importance of taking seriously your diabetes management—you'll get used to it after a while, but you never know what might happen. This is one of the reasons that getting on something like the DASH diet and controlling your blood sugar and other risk factors is so important.

How the DASH diet helps manage diabetes

Okay, now that you have a better understanding of what diabetes is, I can start explaining why the DASH diet is one of the best tools for both preventing type 2 diabetes and managing a pre-existing case of type 2 diabetes.

WebMD discusses three different strategies for diabetics using their diet to help manage the condition:

- increasing fiber intake;
- decreasing fat intake;
- decreasing salt intake.

Does that sound familiar? That's exactly what the DASH diet does. The increased fiber slows the absorption of sugar into your bloodstream, helping to prevent very quick rises in blood sugar. Lowering the amount of fat that you eat helps reduce your risk of heart disease, which can be increased by having diabetes. And eating less salt helps you stave off high blood pressure, which you're also more likely to experience if you have type 2 diabetes.

By focusing on complex carbohydrates (which are high in fiber), fresh fruits and vegetables, and limited but smart meat choices, the DASH diet helps create the perfect strategy for managing your diabetes.

Things to keep in mind when using the DASH diet for diabetes

While the general guidelines of the diet are great for diabetics, there are a few important things to keep in mind if you're using the DASH diet to manage your diabetes. Most importantly, the diet is very flexible, which is generally very advantageous—but if you're dealing with type 2 diabetes, you have to be more careful. For example, if a person with high blood pressure has an item very high on the glycemic index, they'll probably be okay—it might put them over their calorie count for the day, but it probably won't cause health problems if it's not a regular thing. If you're dealing with a serious case of type 2 diabetes, however, making a bad choice could cause problems that you'll need to deal with very quickly. So keep in mind that, although the diet is pretty flexible, you need to stay focused on managing your disease by sticking more closely to the general diabetes treatment guidelines.

The second thing you need to keep in mind is that if you're managing diabetes, you have to think carefully about what you're going to eat, when you're going to eat it, and how much of it you'll have. While I wouldn't recommend it, a person using the DASH diet to curb their blood pressure could probably eat a small breakfast, a small lunch, and a very large dinner, and they'd be fine, as long as they stick to the serving guidelines for the day. If you're diabetic, however, the choices you make throughout the day will affect your blood sugar levels. Let's look at an example. For breakfast, you could eat Rice Krispies and a piece of white toast. This would be two or more servings of carbohydrates, which seems to be fine according to the DASH plan. However, both of these are relatively simple carbohydrates that will raise your blood sugar quickly, and also cause it to fall quickly shortly after. What could you do to make a better choice? You could have a whole-grain cereal, something like Fiber One, a cup of diced fruit instead of toast, and a slice of deli meat or some other lean source of protein. The fiber in the cereal and fruit and the protein in the meat slow down the absorption of sugar, helping you maintain a much more steady blood sugar level.

Eating a larger number of smaller meals (like five or six) throughout the day will also help prevent blood sugar swings.

Finally, I'll re-emphasize the importance of exercise here. No matter what you're using the DASH diet for, exercise is a crucial component. This is especially true of DASH for diabetes, as exercise lowers blood sugar, helping you avoid a hyperglycemic state. You should check your blood sugar before you exercise—if it's looking a little low, it's a good idea to have a small snack before you start your workout.

Notes on exercise before diabetics

If you're a diabetic and you're going to use exercise as part of your treatment plan (or even if you just like to exercise every once in a while), there are some precautions that you should take.

First, as I mentioned, make sure that your blood sugar isn't too low before you start your exercise. If it's lower than it should be (check with your doctor to determine an acceptable measurement), have a small carbohydrate-based snack before you start. It's also a good idea to have some fast-acting carbohydrate snacks with you if you're going to be exercising for more than 30 minutes. Things like glucose tablets, saltine crackers, apple or orange juice, or hard candies like Jolly Ranchers or LifeSavers are all good options. If you start to feel like your blood sugar is dipping too low (if you start to feel dizzy or mentally sluggish, for example), take one of these immediately.

Second, take a measurement of your blood sugar when you're done exercising and have a snack if it's approaching the danger zone. Even if you're done exercising, your blood sugar levels can still be changing, so it's good to keep an eye on them after you're done.

Finally, wear some sort of ID that identifies you as a diabetic. Whether that's a medical alert bracelet, a RoadID, or something like an identification card, it's important that people know that you're diabetic in case of an emergency. Proper treatment can be the difference between life and death in dire situations, so make sure that anyone who might be helping you knows about your condition!

A sample DASH diet plan

You'll notice that this sample plan is quite similar to the others that I've presented before, but that it has one major difference: the sizes of the meals. In the previous plans, there are three meals and three smaller snacks. However, in an effort to keep your blood sugar more stable, your caloric intake (which, in this example, is around 2,000 calories per day) is split more evenly between the meals and snacks. Other than that, it functions on the same principles.

- Breakfast: 2 oz. dry cereal, 8 oz. milk, and 1 cup diced fruit.
- Morning snack: 1/4 cup dried fruit, 1/2 English muffin, and 2 Tbsp. peanut butter.
- Lunch: 1/2 cup cooked potatoes, 1 cup salad, 1 Tbsp. low-fat salad dressing, and 4 oz. fruit juice.
- Afternoon snack: 1 small piece of fruit, 1 oz. cheese, and 6 oz. vegetable juice.
- Dinner: 2/3 cup whole-wheat pasta, 1 oz. lean meat, and 1 cup cooked vegetables.
- Evening snack: 1/2 cup cottage cheese, 1 oz. sliced deli meat, and 1/4 cup canned fruit.

Eating out while on the DASH diet

It may seem a bit strange to dedicate an entire chapter to this subject, but it's one that comes up all the time when discussing the diet. It's always difficult to maintain your diet if you go out to a restaurant or a dinner party, but it can be even more difficult with the DASH diet because of the salt restrictions. So I'll be providing strategies for various courses and meals to help you make it through the day without going over your recommended salt intake as well as reducing the amount of unhealthy fats that you consume.

While these strategies will help you reduce the amount of salt and unhealthy fats that you consume when eating out, it's a good idea to remember that it's still going to be quite difficult to keep your caloric intake to a reasonable level if you're going out to eat. Portion sizes at restaurants are huge (and seem to only get bigger), and it can be very difficult to gauge the number of calories that you're consuming at a meal that you haven't prepared yourself. So even though these are helpful tips, it's still a good idea to minimize the number of times that you eat out on a regular basis.

Breakfast

One of the biggest offenders in the foods-that-aren't-as-healthy-as-most-people-think category is one of my personal favorite breakfast foods: bagels. That's right—even though they're often touted as being healthy breakfast choices, even plain bagels are almost always loaded with salt. And if you indulge in a breakfast sandwich on a bagel, even if it's just eggs and vegetables, you're likely looking at even more salt. So you'll just have to pass.

But bagels aren't the only culprits—other pastries, breakfast meats, and quite a few breakfast cereals are also often high in sodium. Coffee sweeteners are another place that you'll find more sodium than you expected. Be sure to read up on nutrition facts before making your breakfast decisions, or you might find that you've almost reached your daily sodium limit by the time you've finished your first meal!

When it comes to fats, the best strategy you can use is to skip breakfast meats; especially when you're eating out, sausage, bacon, and similar meats are quite unlikely to be lean cuts, and you'll almost certainly be consuming quite a bit of saturated fat from them. Go with eggs instead, and make sure you're getting enough fiber to keep you full until your morning snack. Again, stay away from donuts and pastries, as many of them contain high levels of trans fats.

1. Cottage Cheese Deviled Eggs

Servings: 4

Preparation time: 30 minutes

Cook time: 10 minutes

Ready in: 40 minutes

Nutrition Facts

Serving Size 54 g

Amount Per Serving

Calories 72	Calories from Fat 42

% Daily Value*

Total Fat 4.7g	**7%**
Saturated Fat 1.1g	**5%**
Trans Fat 0.0g	
Cholesterol 105mg	**35%**
Sodium 170mg	**7%**
Total Carbohydrates 1.8g	**1%**
Sugars 0.7g	
Protein 5.8g	

Vitamin A 3%	•	Vitamin C 0%
Calcium 2%	•	Iron 2%

Nutrition Grade C+

* Based on a 2000 calorie diet

Ingredients
- 2 hardboiled egg yolks
- 2 tablespoon Balsamic Vinaigrette
- 1 tablespoon Bac-os Bacon Flavor Chips
- 1 tablespoon 30% Less Sodium, 2% Milkfat Cottage Cheese
- 1/2 tablespoon green onions, chopped
- 4 hardboiled egg whites

Directions
1. **Mash** together the hardboiled egg yolks, vinaigrette, Bac-os, and cheese in a bowl.
2. **Sprinkle** with green onions and blend well.

3. **Fill** the 4 egg white halves with the yolk mixture and chill until serving.

2. Healthy Oatmeal Pancakes

Servings: 4

Preparation time: 10 minutes

Cook time: 10 minutes

Ready in: 20 minutes

Nutrition Facts

Serving Size 104 g

Amount Per Serving

Calories 217   Calories from Fat 81

                         % Daily Value*

Total Fat 9.0g	**14%**
Saturated Fat 1.5g	**7%**
Cholesterol 42mg	**14%**
Sodium 40mg	**2%**
Total Carbohydrates 29.7g	**10%**
Dietary Fiber 1.5g	**6%**
Sugars 8.5g	
Protein 5.9g	

Vitamin A 3%	•	Vitamin C 0%
Calcium 24%	•	Iron 10%

Nutrition Grade B+

* Based on a 2000 calorie diet

Ingredients

- 1/2 cup Whole Wheat flour
- 1/2 cup Quick Cooking oats
- 2 tablespoon Maple syrup
- 3 teaspoon Baking powder
- 3/4 cup Fat-free milk
- 2 tablespoons Olive oil
- 1 egg

Directions

1. **Puree** flour, oats, Maple syrup, baking powder, milk, oil and egg in a food processor until smooth.

2. **Heat** olive oil in a frying pan over medium high heat. Scoop ¼ cup of the batter onto the pan. Lightly brown on both sides.

3. **Serve** with additional syrup or butter on top.

3. Pineapple Carrot Oatmeal Muffins

Servings: 18

Preparation time: 20 minutes

Cook time: 25 minutes

Ready in: 45 minutes

Nutrition Facts

Serving Size 79 g

Amount Per Serving

Calories 216	Calories from Fat 104

% Daily Value*

Total Fat 11.6g	**18%**
Saturated Fat 1.7g	**8%**
Trans Fat 0.0g	
Cholesterol 0mg	**0%**
Sodium 47mg	**2%**
Total Carbohydrates 26.6g	**9%**
Dietary Fiber 1.8g	**7%**
Sugars 11.6g	
Protein 3.6g	

Vitamin A 42%	•	Vitamin C 7%
Calcium 12%	•	Iron 6%

Nutrition Grade C+

* Based on a 2000 calorie diet

Ingredients

- 1 cup All-Purpose flour
- 1 cup Whole Wheat flour
- 3 tablespoons Baking powder
- 1 teaspoon Cinnamon
- 3/4 cup Agave Nectar *
- 1 cup Olive oil
- 6 egg white, beaten
- 1 teaspoon Vanilla extract
- 1/2 cup Uncooked Rolled oats
- 2 cups Carrots, shredded
- 3/4 cup chopped Pineapple
- 1/8 cup Fresh Pineapple juice

- 1/4 cup Fat Free Cream Cheese

Directions

1. **Preheat** oven over 350 degrees F (175 degrees C).
2. **Mix** all-purpose flour, whole wheat flour, baking powder, and cinnamon in a large shallow bowl. Make a hole in the center of the flour mixture, and then add agave nectar, oil, egg white, and vanilla. Whisk just until even. Add in the oats, carrots, and pineapple. Set batter aside.
3. **Combine** the reserved pineapple juice and cream cheese. Fill each muffin cup about 1/2 full with the muffin batter, reserving about 1/3 of the batter. Spoon approximately 1 teaspoon of the cream cheese mixture into the muffin cups. Top with remaining batter, so that each muffin cup is about 2/3 full.
4. **Bake** for about 25 minutes in the preheated oven, or until a toothpick inserted in the center of a muffin comes out clean.

* When baking with agave, honey, or molasses, lower the oven temperature by 25 degrees to avoid overbrowning.

4. Homemade Turkey Patties

Servings: 5

Preparation time: 10 minutes

Cook time: 15 minutes

Ready in: 25 minutes

Nutrition Facts

Serving Size 101 g

Amount Per Serving

Calories 233 Calories from Fat 112

% Daily Value*

Total Fat 12.5g	**19%**
Saturated Fat 2.7g	**14%**
Cholesterol 67mg	**22%**
Sodium 59mg	**2%**
Total Carbohydrates 3.1g	**1%**
Dietary Fiber 0.5g	**2%**
Sugars 2.0g	
Protein 26.3g	

Vitamin A 1%	Vitamin C 1%
Calcium 4%	Iron 9%

Nutrition Grade B-

* Based on a 2000 calorie diet

Ingredients

- 2 teaspoons dried Sage
- 1/2 teaspoon Garlic powder
- 1 teaspoon Onion powder
- 1 teaspoon ground Black Pepper
- 1/4 teaspoon dried Marjoram
- 1 tablespoon Brown sugar
- 1/8 teaspoon crushed Red Pepper flakes
- 1 1/2 teaspoon ground Fennel seed
- 1 pound ground Turkey breast
- 2 tablespoons Olive oil

Directions

1. **Place** the sage, onion powder, garlic powder, ground black pepper, marjoram, brown sugar, red pepper and fennel seed in a large bowl. Mix well to fuse flavors.
2. **Add** the ground turkey in the bowl and using your clean hands combine spices with the turkey. Mix well. Shape spiced ground turkey into round patties.
3. **Warm** olive oil in a large frying pan over medium high heat. Cook both sides of the patties for 5 minutes, or until internal meat reach the temperature of 160 degrees F (73 degrees C).

5. Buttermilk and Chocolate Chip Waffles

Servings: 10

Preparation time: 15 minutes

Cook time: 2 minutes

Ready in: 17 minutes

Nutrition Facts

Serving Size 84 g

Amount Per Serving

Calories 204	Calories from Fat 87

	% Daily Value*
Total Fat 9.6g	**15%**
Saturated Fat 5.7g	**29%**
Trans Fat 0.0g	
Cholesterol 57mg	**19%**
Sodium 45mg	**2%**
Total Carbohydrates 24.2g	**8%**
Dietary Fiber 1.1g	**5%**
Sugars 7.2g	
Protein 4.4g	

Vitamin A 4%	•	Vitamin C 1%
Calcium 12%	•	Iron 6%

Nutrition Grade B-

* Based on a 2000 calorie diet

Ingredients

- 1 1/2 cups Whole Wheat flour
- 1 cup Low-fat buttermilk
- 3 1/4 teaspoons Baking powder
- 1/4 cup Half and Half
- 1/4 cup Fat-free milk
- 2 egg yolks
- 1/4 cup Unsalted Danish Butter, melted
- 2 egg whites
- 1/2 cup Semisweet Chocolate Chips
- Olive oil or coconut oil for greasing

Directions

1. **Mix** the flour, buttermilk, and baking powder in a large bowl. Using electric mixer, whip half and half, milk, egg yolks, and melted butter in a separate bowl. Mix until smooth. Pour the milk mixture into the flour mixture and stir until even. Set aside.

2. **Whip** egg whites to firm peaks in a clean metal bowl. Using a spatula, fold whipped egg whites and chocolate chips into the batter.

3. **Heat** a waffle iron, and drizzle little olive oil. Scoop batter onto the hot waffle iron. Cook until the waffles are lightly browned or there is no longer steam coming out from the iron.

6. Low-fat Banana Nut Bread

Servings: 12

Preparation time: 15 minutes

Cook time: 1 hour

Ready in: 1 hour and 15 minutes

Nutrition Facts

Serving Size 69 g

Amount Per Serving

Calories 146   Calories from Fat 25

                                   % Daily Value*

Total Fat 2.8g   **4%**

   Trans Fat 0.0g

Cholesterol 0mg   **0%**

Sodium 123mg   **5%**

Total Carbohydrates 26.6g   **9%**

   Dietary Fiber 1.5g   **6%**

   Sugars 8.6g

Protein 4.6g

Vitamin A 0%   •   Vitamin C 2%

Calcium 1%   •   Iron 7%

Nutrition Grade A-

* Based on a 2000 calorie diet

Ingredients

- 1/3 cup Unsweetened Applesauce
- 1/4 cup Raw Honey*
- 4 egg whites
- 1 cup mashed Bananas
- 1 teaspoon Maple Syrup
- 1/2 teaspoon ground Cinnamon
- 1/2 teaspoon ground Nutmeg
- 2 cups Whole Wheat flour
- 1 teaspoon Baking soda
- 1/4 cup hot Water
- 1/4 cup Walnuts, chopped
- 1/4 cup Almond, chopped

Directions

1. **Preheat** oven to 325 degrees F (165 degrees C).
2. **Whisk** applesauce and honey together in a bowl. Add egg whites, maple syrup, cinnamon, and nutmeg. Fold in bananas. Mix well.
3. **Stir** in flour. In a ¼ cup hot water add baking soda, stir to mix, and then pour into the batter. Toss in chopped nuts. Cover a greased 9x5 inch loaf pan with the batter.
4. **Bake** into the preheated oven for about 1 hour. Transfer into a wire rack and let cool for about half hour before slicing.

* When baking with agave, honey, or molasses, lower the oven temperature by 25 degrees to avoid overbrowning.

7. Breakfast Brussels and Turkey Bacon

Servings: 6

Preparation time: 15 minutes

Cook time: 15 minutes

Ready in: 30 minutes

Nutrition Facts

Serving Size 107 g

Amount Per Serving

Calories 59	Calories from Fat 7

% Daily Value*

Total Fat 0.8g	**1%**
Trans Fat 0.0g	
Cholesterol 10mg	**3%**
Sodium 143mg	**6%**
Total Carbohydrates 8.2g	**3%**
Dietary Fiber 3.0g	**12%**
Sugars 1.7g	
Protein 5.9g	

Vitamin A 13%	•	Vitamin C 108%
Calcium 4%	•	Iron 7%

Nutrition Grade A

* Based on a 2000 calorie diet

Ingredients

- 6 slices Turkey bacon
- 3 tablespoon Shallots, chopped
- 2 clove Garlic, minced
- 16 oz. fresh Brussels Sprouts, steamed and halved
- 1 teaspoon ground Black Pepper
- 1/4 cup Low Sodium Chicken stock

Directions

1. **Cook** bacon in a large frying pan over medium-high heat and until crisp. Drain oil, reserving 2 teaspoons. Crumble the bacon and set aside.

2. **Reheat** the reserved oil over medium-high heat. Stir in the shallots and garlic in the oil until shallots is translucent. Add the Brussels sprouts and crumbled bacon; cook for 5 minutes, stirring occasionally. Sprinkle with dash of pepper.
3. **Pour** in chicken stock and reduce liquid to half, scraping the browned bits at the bottom of pan. Serve warm.

8. Cheesy Baby Spinach Omelet

Servings: 2

Preparation time: 6 minutes

Cook time: 9 minutes

Ready in: 15 minutes

Nutrition Facts

Serving Size 151 g

Amount Per Serving

Calories 110	Calories from Fat 39

% Daily Value*

Total Fat 4.3g	**7%**
Saturated Fat 2.3g	**12%**
Cholesterol 10mg	**3%**
Sodium 193mg	**8%**
Total Carbohydrates 6.9g	**2%**
Dietary Fiber 1.6g	**6%**
Sugars 2.8g	
Protein 11.8g	

Vitamin A 30%	Vitamin C 16%
Calcium 12%	Iron 3%

Nutrition Grade B

* Based on a 2000 calorie diet

Ingredients

- 4 egg white
- 1 teaspoon Garlic powder
- 1/8 teaspoon ground Nutmeg
- 1/2 teaspoon ground Black Pepper
- 1 Onion, chopped
- 1 cup Baby Spinach
- 2 tablespoon Provolone Cheese - 42% Lower Sodium
- Cooking spray

Directions

1. **Beat** the egg whites, garlic powder, nutmeg, and pepper in a clean metal bowl.

2. **Heat** a small skillet coated with cooking spray over medium heat, toss in onion and cook until softened. Add baby spinach and cheese. Let cheese slightly melted.
3. **Pour** in the egg white mixture and cook about 3 minutes, or until partially set. Flip omelet and cook for another 3 minutes.
4. **Reduce** heat to low, and continue cooking until desire doneness.

9. Walnut, Raisins & Pumpkin Oatmeal

Servings: 2

Preparation time: 5 minutes

Cook time: 10 minutes

Ready in: 15 minutes

Nutrition Facts

Serving Size 136 g

Amount Per Serving

Calories 151	Calories from Fat 47

% Daily Value*

Total Fat 5.2g	**8%**
Saturated Fat 0.5g	**3%**
Trans Fat 0.0g	
Cholesterol 0mg	**0%**
Sodium 78mg	**3%**
Total Carbohydrates 22.8g	**8%**
Dietary Fiber 4.3g	**17%**
Sugars 5.3g	
Protein 4.7g	

Vitamin A 95%	•	Vitamin C 3%
Calcium 3%	•	Iron 9%

Nutrition Grade A

* Based on a 2000 calorie diet

Ingredients

- 1 cup Unsweetened Almond Milk
- 1/4 cup pureed Pumpkin
- 1/2 cup Rolled oats
- 1/2 teaspoon ground Nutmeg
- 1/2 teaspoon ground Cinnamon
- 1 tablespoon chopped Walnuts
- 1 tablespoon Raisin
- 1/2 tablespoon Agave Nectar liquid sweetener

Directions

1. **Pour** almond milk and pumpkin puree in a medium saucepan. Stir in the oats, dash of nutmeg and cinnamon and bring to a boil.
2. **Reduce** the heat to low and simmer oatmeal for 5 minutes, or until it reaches your desired evenness.
3. **Remove** from heat and transfer to serving bowl. Garnish with walnuts, raisins and swirl of agave.

10. Strawberry Rounds

Servings: 8

Preparation time: 10 minutes

Cook time: 3 minutes

Ready in: 13 minutes

Nutrition Facts

Serving Size 67 g

Amount Per Serving

Calories 182 — Calories from Fat 79

% Daily Value*

Total Fat 8.8g	**14%**
Saturated Fat 1.2g	**6%**
Trans Fat 0.0g	
Cholesterol 0mg	**0%**
Sodium 176mg	**7%**
Total Carbohydrates 21.7g	**7%**
Dietary Fiber 3.9g	**16%**
Sugars 7.7g	
Protein 7.0g	

Vitamin A 2% • Vitamin C 10%
Calcium 10% • Iron 7%

Nutrition Grade A-
* Based on a 2000 calorie diet

Ingredients

- 1/2 cup unsalted Peanut Butter
- 4 Whole Wheat English muffins, halved and toasted
- ½ cup strawberry, sliced
- 1/8 cup Pure Agave Nectar
- 2 tablespoons Trans-fat free Margarine, melted
- 1/4 teaspoon ground Cinnamon

Directions

1. **Spread** a tablespoon of peanut butter onto each muffin half. Place strawberry slices on top of each one.
2. **Whip** agave, margarine, and cinnamon until even. Drizzle the agave mixture over strawberry slices and serve.

11. Cheesy Crust less Spinach, Onion and Mushroom Quiche

Servings: 6

Preparation time: 20 minutes

Cook time: 25 minutes

Ready in: 45 minutes

Nutrition Facts

Serving Size 154 g

Amount Per Serving

Calories 117   Calories from Fat 65

       % Daily Value*

	% Daily Value*
Total Fat 7.3g	11%
Saturated Fat 1.5g	8%
Trans Fat 0.0g	
Cholesterol 5mg	2%
Sodium 164mg	7%
Total Carbohydrates 7.1g	2%
Dietary Fiber 1.5g	6%
Sugars 4.1g	
Protein 7.8g	

Vitamin A 58%	•	Vitamin C 17%
Calcium 13%	•	Iron 7%

Nutrition Grade A

* Based on a 2000 calorie diet

Ingredients

- 2 tablespoon Olive oil
- 1 medium Onion, diced
- 6 Oz fresh Baby Spinach
- 1/2 cup fresh Mushroom, sliced
- 5 egg whites
- 1/2 cup Almond flour
- 1/2 teaspoon Baking powder
- 1/2 teaspoon cayenne pepper
- 1 teaspoon Black Pepper, ground

- 1/2 teaspoon Garlic powder
- 1 1/3 cups Low-fat milk
- 1/4 cup Low-fat feta cheese

Directions

1. **Preheat** oven to 400F (200 degrees C).
2. **Grease** with 1 tablespoon of olive oil a 10-inch quiche pan. Heat remaining olive oil over medium-high heat in a medium frying pan.
3. **Stir** in onion and cook until softened. Toss in baby spinach and mushrooms. Cook until just wilted. Set aside.
4. **Whisk** together eggs, flour, baking powder, cayenne, pepper and garlic powder in a large mixing bowl. Pour in milk and whisk to combine. Fold in spinach mixture. Pour mixture into the quiche pan. Top with crumbled feta cheese.
5. **Bake** until center is set and the outside edge is crisp brown, about 25 minutes.
6. **Remove** from oven and let set for about 5 minutes. Slice and serve.

12. Easy Tuna Salad

Servings: 4

Preparation time: 15 minutes

Cook time: 15 minutes

Ready in: 30 minutes

Nutrition Facts

Serving Size 121 g

Amount Per Serving

Calories 79   Calories from Fat 4

	% Daily Value*
Total Fat 0.4g	**1%**
Trans Fat 0.0g	
Cholesterol 17mg	**6%**
Sodium 85mg	**4%**
Total Carbohydrates 6.4g	**2%**
Dietary Fiber 1.1g	**4%**
Sugars 3.9g	
Protein 10.7g	

Vitamin A 5%   •   Vitamin C 10%
Calcium 6%   •   Iron 3%

Nutrition Grade B+

* Based on a 2000 calorie diet

Ingredients

- 1/2 cup Low-fat plain Yogurt
- 6 Oz canned Tuna, drained
- 1/4 cup Celery, chopped
- 1 large Yellow Onion
- 1/2 teaspoon Garlic powder
- 1/2 teaspoon ground black pepper
- 1/2 teaspoon Paprika
- 1/2 teaspoon Lemon juice
- 1 tablespoon fresh Parsley, chopped

Directions

1. **Place** yogurt in a large deep bowl. Add tuna, celery, onion, garlic powder, pepper, paprika and lemon juice. Mix well to combine flavors.

2. **Sprinkle** the top with some freshly chopped parsley. Refrigerate until chilled.

13. Vegetable Egg-white Scrambled

Servings: 6

Preparation time: 10 minutes

Cook time: 15 minutes

Ready in: 25 minutes

Nutrition Facts

Serving Size 161 g

Amount Per Serving

Calories 137 — Calories from Fat 81

% Daily Value*

Total Fat 9.0g	**14%**
Saturated Fat 1.4g	**7%**
Trans Fat 0.0g	
Cholesterol 1mg	**0%**
Sodium 120mg	**5%**
Total Carbohydrates 7.5g	**2%**
Dietary Fiber 1.9g	**8%**
Sugars 4.6g	
Protein 7.4g	

Vitamin A 38%	•	Vitamin C 133%
Calcium 3%	•	Iron 3%

Nutrition Grade B

* Based on a 2000 calorie diet

Ingredients

- 1/4 cup Olive oil
- 1/4 cup Portabella Mushroom, sliced
- 1 large Yellow Onion, chopped
- 1 Green Bell Pepper, chopped
- 1 Red Bell Pepper, chopped
- 1 Yellow Bell Pepper, chopped
- 8 egg whites
- 1/4 cup Low-fat Cottage cheese
- 1/4 cup Low Fat Milk
- 1/4 cup fresh Tomato, chopped
- 2 tablespoon fresh Cilantro, chopped

Directions

1. **Warm** olive oil in a skillet over medium-high heat. Sauté mushrooms, onions and peppers until onions are translucent.
2. **Beat** together egg whites, cheese and milk in a bowl. Pour egg mixture to vegetables and toss in tomatoes. Cook until eggs are well done.
3. **Sprinkle** with chopped cilantro and serve.

14. Cinnamon Apples in Nutty Quinoa Porridge

Servings: 3

Preparation time: 10 minutes

Cook time: 30 minutes

Ready in: 40 minutes

Nutrition Facts

Serving Size 334 g

Amount Per Serving

Calories 503   Calories from Fat 276

                 % Daily Value*

	% Daily Value*
Total Fat 30.7g	**47%**
Saturated Fat 21.1g	**105%**
Trans Fat 0.0g	
Cholesterol 8mg	**3%**
Sodium 18mg	**1%**
Total Carbohydrates 53.3g	**18%**
Dietary Fiber 8.1g	**32%**
Sugars 18.6g	
Protein 10.1g	

Vitamin A 2%   •   Vitamin C 6%

Calcium 9%   •   Iron 22%

Nutrition Grade C

* Based on a 2000 calorie diet

Ingredients

- 1 cup Red Quinoa, rinsed and drained
- 2 cups Water
- 1 tablespoon Unsalted Butter
- 1 Pink Lady Apple, peeled, cored and diced
- 1 tablespoon ground Cinnamon
- 2 tablespoons Maple Syrup
- 1/3 cup toasted Almond, chopped
- 1 1/2 cups Coconut Milk

Directions

1. **Place** water in a large saucepan over high heat. Add quinoa and bring to boil. Reduce heat to medium-low, cover the saucepan, and simmer for 20 minutes, or until the quinoa is soft and the water has been soaked up. Remove from heat and set aside.
2. **Melt** butter in a large pan over medium heat. Add the apple, cinnamon, and maple syrup. Toss in the almonds. Cook and stir for about 3 minutes, or until the apple begins to soften.
3. **Pour** in the coconut milk and continue cooking until liquid is boiling. Stir in the quinoa. Cook for a minute or two, just before serving.

Lunch

Just like many breakfast foods, a lot of things that people often think of as healthy lunch choices can pack quite a bit of salt. You might already be aware that pre-packaged meals (even some of those from such low-calorie brands as Weight Watchers and Lean Cuisine) can pack a lot of salt into a single serving. But do you know how much salt is in the bread, meat, and cheese that come with your sandwich from the local deli? I'd recommend finding out, because it could be a lot more than you bargained for

If you're being disciplined and eating a salad for lunch, good job! But be careful about the dressing you use—bottled salad dressings can be really high in sodium. A better alternative is to use an oil-and-vinegar mix or just a tiny splash of bottled vinaigrette. In general, condiments are pretty high in sodium, so go really light on the ketchup, mustard, and mayo, too.

If you go out for lunch, you might be tempted to order something that includes meat, and that's okay—if you're careful about which meat you choose. Opting for meats that have been prepared with healthier methods, like grilling, broiling, baking, and roasting, is going to help you more than if you choose one that's been fried or smoked. You can always ask that your food be prepared with olive oil instead of butter or vegetable oil—that won't help your overall calorie intake much, but it will help you avoid unhealthy fats.

1. Sweet and Tangy Cranberry Spinach Salad

Servings: 4

Preparation time: 10 minutes

Cook time: 15 minutes

Ready in: 25 minutes

Nutrition Facts

Serving Size 245 g

Amount Per Serving

Calories 475	Calories from Fat 353

	% Daily Value*
Total Fat 39.2g	**60%**
Saturated Fat 5.7g	**28%**
Trans Fat 0.0g	
Cholesterol 0mg	**0%**
Sodium 108mg	**4%**
Total Carbohydrates 29.0g	**10%**
Dietary Fiber 6.6g	**26%**
Sugars 18.6g	
Protein 8.6g	

Vitamin A 214%	•	Vitamin C 59%
Calcium 24%	•	Iron 26%

Nutrition Grade B

* Based on a 2000 calorie diet

Ingredients

- 1 tablespoon Low-fat Butter
- 3/4 cup Almonds, peeled and chopped
- 2 tablespoons Sesame Seeds, toasted
- 1 tablespoon Poppy Seeds
- 1/4 cup Raw Agave Nectar
- 2 teaspoons Onion, minced
- 1/4 teaspoon Paprika
- 1/4 cup Balsamic Vinegar
- 1/4 cup Cider Vinegar
- 1/2 cup Olive oil
- 1 pound Spinach, torn
- 1 cup Cranberries, halved

Directions

1. **Soften** the butter in a medium saucepan over medium heat. Toast almonds in butter until browned. Remove from heat, and set aside.
2. **Whisk** together the sesame seeds, poppy seeds, sugar, onion, paprika, white wine vinegar, cider vinegar, and vegetable oil in a large mixing bowl.
3. **Toss** in spinach, toasted almonds and cranberries. Serve.

2. Crispy Fish Cabbage Tacos

Servings: 3

Preparation time: 40 minutes

Cook time: 20 minutes

Ready in: 1 hour

Nutrition Facts

Serving Size 546 g

Amount Per Serving

Calories 612   Calories from Fat 318

% **Daily Value***

Total Fat 35.3g	**54%**
Saturated Fat 5.0g	**25%**
Trans Fat 0.0g	
Cholesterol 28mg	**9%**
Sodium 226mg	**9%**
Total Carbohydrates 52.6g	**18%**
Dietary Fiber 8.4g	**34%**
Sugars 18.2g	
Protein 26.9g	

Vitamin A 12%   •   Vitamin C 153%

Calcium 28%   •   Iron 17%

Nutrition Grade B

* Based on a 2000 calorie diet

Ingredients

- 1/2 cup All-purpose Flour
- 1/2 teaspoon Baking Powder
- 2 egg white
- 1/2 cup Apple Cider
- 1 cup Non-fat Yogurt
- 1 tablespoon Lime juice
- 1 Jalapeno Pepper, minced
- 1 teaspoon Capers, minced
- 1/2 teaspoon fresh Cilantro, chopped
- 1/2 teaspoon ground Cumin
- 1/2 teaspoon fresh Dill, minced
- 1/2 teaspoon Cayenne, ground

- 1/2 cup Olive Oil
- 8 Oz Cod Fillets, slice into thick strips
- 3 Corn Tortillas
- 1 head Red Cabbage, shredded

Directions

Apple cider batter:

1. **Beat** egg whites, apple cider, flour and baking powder in a large bowl (don't worry about a few lumps).

White sauce:

1. **Place** yogurt in a medium mixing bowl. Slowly stir in fresh lime juice until sauce is slightly runny. Add jalapeno, capers, cilantro, cumin, dill, and cayenne. Mix well.
2. **Preheat** oil in deep-fryer to 375 degrees F (190 degrees C).
3. **Dust** cod strips lightly with flour. Dip it into the apple cider batter. Fry until crispy and golden. Drain excess oil onto paper towels.
4. **Fry** tortillas until just crisp. Place two cod strips in each tortilla, top with cabbage, and drizzle white sauce.

3. Tuna, Onion and Tomato in Pita Bread

Servings: 6

Preparation time: 10 minutes

Cook time: 10 minutes

Ready in: 20 minutes

Nutrition Facts

Serving Size 223 g

Amount Per Serving

Calories 368   Calories from Fat 104

% Daily Value*

Total Fat 11.6g	**18%**
Saturated Fat 5.0g	**25%**
Cholesterol 37mg	**12%**
Sodium 509mg	**21%**
Total Carbohydrates 38.7g	**13%**
Dietary Fiber 2.2g	**9%**
Sugars 4.0g	
Protein 25.8g	

Vitamin A 6%   •   Vitamin C 14%
Calcium 19%   •   Iron 15%

Nutrition Grade B

* Based on a 2000 calorie diet

Ingredients

- 6 Pitas, 6-inch
- 12 Oz Tuna in can, drained
- 2 tablespoons Non-fat Mayonnaise
- 2 tablespoons Dill Pickle Relish
- 1/4 teaspoon Black Pepper, ground
- 1 teaspoon Garlic powder
- 1 white Onion, sliced into wedges
- 1 large tomato, sliced into wedges
- 1 cup shredded Low-fat Cheddar cheese

Directions

1. **Preheat** the oven to 400 degrees F (200 degrees C).
2. **Combine** together the tuna, mayonnaise, relish, pepper and garlic powder. Mix well. Set aside.
3. **Place** pita breads in a single layer on a baking dish. Bake in the preheated oven for 5 minutes, or until lightly crisp.
4. **Cover** each pita bread with equal amount of the tuna mixture. Top the tuna with onions and tomato wedges, and then sprinkle with shredded cheese.
5. **Return** pita breads into the preheated oven and bake for 5 minutes, or until cheese has melted.

4. Tropical Scallop Ceviche

Servings: 4

Preparation time: 20 minutes

Cook time: 2 hours and 10 minutes

Ready in: 2 hours and 30 minutes

Nutrition Facts

Serving Size 346 g

Amount Per Serving

Calories 219	Calories from Fat 14

	% Daily Value*
Total Fat 1.6g	**2%**
Cholesterol 37mg	**12%**
Sodium 187mg	**8%**
Total Carbohydrates 35.0g	**12%**
Dietary Fiber 6.1g	**24%**
Sugars 21.4g	
Protein 20.9g	

Vitamin A 22%	•	Vitamin C 153%
Calcium 8%	•	Iron 6%

Nutrition Grade A

* Based on a 2000 calorie diet

Ingredients

- 1 pound Sea Scallops, trimmed and halved
- 2 ripe mangoes, peeled and chopped
- 4 Lime, juiced
- 1 Orange, juiced
- 1/3 cup Red onion, thinly sliced
- 1 Poblanos Pepper, thinly sliced
- 1 teaspoon Black Pepper, ground
- 4 Romaine Leaves

Directions

1. **Simmer** scallops into a 1/2 inch water in a large skillet over medium heat and cook until firm, about 3 to 5 minutes. Remove from heat and drain the scallops using a slotted spoon. Transfer scallop into a clean medium bowl.
2. **Toss** half of the mango into the bowl with the scallops. Blend the remaining mango with lime juice and orange juice in a blender until even.
3. **Pour** puree over the scallops and chunks of mango. Add poblanos peppers and onion. Gently mix to incorporate flavors. Season with dash of pepper. Cover and let the ceviche chill for 2 hours. Serve.

5. Broccoli and Chicken Pasta

Servings: 6

Preparation time: 10 minutes

Cook time: 20 minutes

Ready in: 30 minutes

Nutrition Facts

Serving Size 210 g

Amount Per Serving

Calories 419   Calories from Fat 144

                                         % Daily Value*

Total Fat 16.0g	**25%**
Saturated Fat 4.2g	**21%**
Trans Fat 0.0g	
Cholesterol 117mg	**39%**
Sodium 211mg	**9%**
Total Carbohydrates 35.6g	**12%**
Dietary Fiber 1.4g	**6%**
Sugars 1.6g	
Protein 33.0g	

Vitamin A 7%   •   Vitamin C 54%

Calcium 14%   •   Iron 20%

Nutrition Grade B+

* Based on a 2000 calorie diet

Ingredients

- 12 ounces Rigatoni Pasta
- 2 cups fresh Broccoli Florets
- 2 tablespoon Olive oil
- 1 tablespoon Garlic, minced
- 1 tablespoon Onion, chopped
- 2 tablespoons Pesto
- 1 cup Tomatoes, chopped
- 1 teaspoon dried Oregano
- 1 pound boneless skinless Chicken Breast, cooked and clunked
- 2 Oz Parmesan Cheese, shredded
- 1 teaspoon Black Pepper, ground

Directions

1. **Bring** water to boil in a large pot. Cook rigatoni pasta until well done. Remove and drain.
2. **Blanch** broccoli florets in a medium saucepan over medium-high heat. Remove from pan using a slotted spoon.
3. **Heat** olive oil in the saucepan over medium- high heat. Stir in garlic, onion and pesto sauce for 2 minutes. Add tomatoes and oregano. Cook and set aside.
4. **Combine** pasta, broccoli, cooked chicken, and pesto mix in a large mixing bowl. Top pasta mix with grated Parmesan cheese, and dash of ground black pepper. Serve warm.

6. Herbs and Tomato Soup

Servings: 4

Preparation time: 5 minutes

Cook time: 30 minutes

Ready in: 35 minutes

Nutrition Facts

Serving Size 292 g

Amount Per Serving

Calories 100   Calories from Fat 32

	% Daily Value*
Total Fat 3.6g	**5%**
Saturated Fat 1.9g	**10%**
Cholesterol 0mg	**0%**
Sodium 74mg	**3%**
Total Carbohydrates 14.9g	**5%**
Dietary Fiber 2.9g	**11%**
Sugars 7.0g	
Protein 3.7g	

Vitamin A 7%   •   Vitamin C 57%
Calcium 3%   •   Iron 22%

Nutrition Grade A-
* Based on a 2000 calorie diet

Ingredients

- 2 cups Low Sodium Chicken Broth
- 4 cups fresh Tomatoes, chopped
- 1 tablespoon chopped Onion
- 4 cloves Garlic, crushed
- 1 Bay Leaf
- 1 teaspoon Cayenne, ground
- 1 tablespoon dried Oregano
- 1 teaspoon Thyme
- 30g Low Fat Butter
- 2 tablespoons All-purpose Flour
- 2 teaspoons Raw Honey

Directions

1. **Pour** chicken broth into a stockpot over medium heat. Add the tomatoes, onion, garlic, bay leaf, cayenne, oregano, and thyme. Gently bring to boil for about 20 minutes to let flavors to blend.
2. **Remove** mixture from heat and pass through a food mill into a large bowl, and then discard left over in the food mill.
3. **Melt** the butter in a shallow stockpot over medium heat. Add in the flour to make a roux, and cook until lightly brown. Slowly whisk in the tomato mixture, so no lumps will form. Add honey for little sweetness.

7. Oven Roast Vegetables

Servings: 12

Preparation time: 15 minutes

Cook time: 40 minutes

Ready in: 55 minutes

Nutrition Facts

Serving Size 123 g

Amount Per Serving

Calories 91   Calories from Fat 40

	% Daily Value*
Total Fat 4.5g	**7%**
Saturated Fat 0.7g	**3%**
Trans Fat 0.0g	
Cholesterol 0mg	**0%**
Sodium 89mg	**4%**
Total Carbohydrates 11.9g	**4%**
Dietary Fiber 2.1g	**8%**
Sugars 1.9g	
Protein 1.8g	

Vitamin A 15%	•	Vitamin C 82%
Calcium 2%	•	Iron 5%

Nutrition Grade A

* Based on a 2000 calorie diet

Ingredients

- 1 small Zucchini, cubed
- 2 Red Bell peppers, diced
- 3 Yukon Gold Potatoes, cubed
- 2 cups Broccoli Florets
- 8 Oz Cherry Tomato, halved and seeded
- 1 Red Onion, quartered and separated into pieces
- 2 teaspoon fresh Thyme
- 1 tablespoon fresh Rosemary
- 1/4 cup Extra Virgin Olive Oil
- 2 tablespoons Balsamic Vinegar
- ½ teaspoon Sea Salt
- 1 teaspoon Black Pepper, crushed

Directions

1. **Preheat** oven to 475 degrees F (245 degrees C).
2. **Place** zucchini together with red bell peppers, potatoes, broccoli, cherry tomato, and onion in a large bowl.
3. **Mix** together thyme, rosemary, olive oil, vinegar, salt, and pepper in a small bowl. Toss with vegetables until well coated. Scatter vegetables on a large roasting pan.
4. **Roast** vegetables into the oven for 35 to 40 minutes, or until browned and cooked through, stirring every 10 minutes.

8. Veggies and Turkey Stew

Servings: 4-5

Preparation time: 15 minutes

Cook time: 50 minutes

Ready in: 1 hour and 5 minutes

Nutrition Facts

Serving Size 382 g

Amount Per Serving

Calories 219	Calories from Fat 43

% Daily Value*

Total Fat 4.8g	**7%**
Trans Fat 0.0g	
Cholesterol 39mg	**13%**
Sodium 107mg	**4%**
Total Carbohydrates 25.0g	**8%**
Dietary Fiber 4.3g	**17%**
Sugars 5.0g	
Protein 18.7g	

Vitamin A 41%	•	Vitamin C 137%
Calcium 2%	•	Iron 10%

Nutrition Grade A

* Based on a 2000 calorie diet

Ingredients

- 1 tablespoon Olive Oil
- 2 Onions, chopped
- 2 Potatoes, cubed
- 1 Celery stalk, sliced
- 2 Baby Carrots, sliced
- 3 tablespoons All-purpose flour
- 3 cups Low Sodium Chicken stock
- 1/4 teaspoon dried Marjoram
- 1 teaspoon fresh Rosemary
- 8 Oz Chicken Breast, skinless, boneless, cubed
- 1 Green Bell Pepper, diced
- 1 Red Bell Pepper, diced

Directions

1. **Warm** olive oil in a pot over medium heat. Stir in onions and cook until softened. Toss in potatoes, celery and carrots, and cook until tender. Add some flour.
2. **Pour** in the chicken stock, and season with marjoram and rosemary. Place turkey in the pot, and bring to a boil. Reduce heat to low, and then simmer for 30 minutes.
3. **Add** the bell peppers and continue cooking for 10 more minutes.

9. Fruits and Chicken Salad

Servings: 10

Preparation time: 15 minutes

Cook time: 15 minutes

Ready in: 30 minutes

Nutrition Facts

Serving Size 109 g

Amount Per Serving

Calories 207	Calories from Fat 122

	% Daily Value*
Total Fat 13.6g	**21%**
Saturated Fat 2.2g	**11%**
Trans Fat 0.0g	
Cholesterol 43mg	**14%**
Sodium 253mg	**11%**
Total Carbohydrates 9.2g	**3%**
Dietary Fiber 1.7g	**7%**
Sugars 3.5g	
Protein 14.5g	

Vitamin A 5%	•	Vitamin C 9%
Calcium 2%	•	Iron 3%

Nutrition Grade C+

* Based on a 2000 calorie diet

Ingredients

- 1 pound Rotisserie Chicken, shredded
- 1/2 cup Low-fat Whipping Cream
- 1/2 cup Low-fat Mayonnaise
- 1 Lemon, juiced
- 1 teaspoon paprika
- 1/2 cup dried Cranberries
- 1/2 cup dried Cherry
- 1/2 cup Green Grapes, halved
- 1/2 cup Apple, chopped
- 2 stalk Celery, chopped
- 2 Green Onions, chopped
- 1 cup toasted Walnuts, chopped

- 1 dash of ground Black Pepper

Directions

1. **Mix** together whipping cream, mayonnaise, lemon juice, and paprika in a large mixing bowl.
2. **Toss** in dried cranberries, cherry, grapes, apple, celery, green onions, and nuts. Add rotisserie chicken, and mix well. Season with black pepper to taste.
3. **Chill** for 1 hour before serving.

10. Savory Beef with Vegetables Stir-fry

Servings: 4

Preparation time: 10 minutes

Cook time: 30 minutes

Ready in: 40 minutes

Nutrition Facts

Serving Size 321 g

Amount Per Serving

Calories 240   Calories from Fat 98

	% Daily Value*
Total Fat 10.9g	**17%**
Saturated Fat 2.4g	**12%**
Trans Fat 0.0g	
Cholesterol 51mg	**17%**
Sodium 202mg	**8%**
Total Carbohydrates 14.3g	**5%**
Dietary Fiber 3.2g	**13%**
Sugars 7.2g	
Protein 20.3g	

Vitamin A 59%   •   Vitamin C 229%
Calcium 2%   •   Iron 65%

Nutrition Grade A
* Based on a 2000 calorie diet

Ingredients

- 8 ounces Beef Sirloin, sliced into strips
- 2 tablespoons Olive oil
- 1 Onion, chopped
- 2 clove Garlic, minced
- 2 teaspoon chopped fresh Ginger Root
- 1 Green Bell Pepper, Julienne cut
- 1 Yellow Bell Pepper, Julienne cut
- 1 Red Bell Pepper, Julienne cut
- 1 cup Broccoli Florets
- 1/2 cup Mushroom, thin sliced
- 1 (10.5 ounce) can Beef broth 50% Less Sodium
- 1 tablespoon Cornstarch

- 1 teaspoon Raw Honey
- 1 tablespoon Coconut aminos
- 15g Dry Sherry
- 1/2 teaspoon Black Pepper, ground

Directions

1. **Sauté** beef slices in the oil for 5 minutes or until browned, in a large skillet over medium high heat. Toss in the onion, garlic and ginger and stir for 5 more minutes.
2. **Add** bell peppers, broccoli, mushrooms and beef broth. Reduce heat to low and let simmer.
3. **Combine** the cornstarch, honey, coconut aminos and dry sherry in a small bowl. Stir thoroughly until smooth.
4. **Gradually** pour to the simmering beef and vegetables, stirring well. Simmer more until desired thickness of the sauce. Sprinkle with a dash of pepper to taste.

11. Dutch Vegetable Curry

Servings: 6

Preparation time: 20 minutes

Cook time: 45 minutes

Ready in: 1 hour and 5 minutes

Nutrition Facts

Serving Size 390 g

Amount Per Serving

Calories 216	Calories from Fat 72

% Daily Value*

Total Fat 8.0g	**12%**
Saturated Fat 2.9g	**15%**
Cholesterol 0mg	**0%**
Sodium 30mg	**1%**
Total Carbohydrates 35.3g	**12%**
Dietary Fiber 7.6g	**30%**
Sugars 8.0g	
Protein 5.5g	

Vitamin A 32%	Vitamin C 169%
Calcium 4%	Iron 22%

Nutrition Grade A

* Based on a 2000 calorie diet

Ingredients

- 2 tablespoons Olive Oil
- 1 White Onion, chopped
- 4 cloves Garlic, Crushed
- 1 tablespoon Curry powder
- 1/2 teaspoon Cumin seeds
- 1 Eggplant, cubed
- 1 Green Bell Pepper, chopped
- 1 Red Bell Pepper, chopped
- 4 Yukon Gold potatoes, chunked
- 3 tomatoes, chopped
- 3 small Zucchini, chopped
- 1/2 teaspoon chili powder

- 1/4 teaspoon Red Pepper flakes
- 1/2 teaspoon ground Turmeric
- 1/4 cup Coconut Milk
- 1/4 cup chopped fresh Coriander
- 1 tablespoon chopped Parsley

Directions

1. **Heat** olive oil in a Dutch oven or large pot over medium heat. Sauté onion and garlic and cook until onion are translucent. Add curry powder and cumin until pungent.
2. **Toss** in eggplant, bell peppers, potatoes, tomatoes, zucchini, chili powder, pepper flakes and turmeric. Pour in coconut milk. Simmer for 30 to 45 minutes; add water to maintain a stew-like consistency, if necessary.
3. **Garnish** with coriander and parsley just before serving.

12. Turkey Salad with Dill Pickle Relish

Servings: 5

Preparation time: 20 minutes

Nutrition Facts

Serving Size 275 g

Amount Per Serving

Calories 314	Calories from Fat 110

% Daily Value*

Total Fat 12.2g	**19%**
Saturated Fat 5.6g	**28%**
Cholesterol 118mg	**39%**
Sodium 255mg	**11%**
Total Carbohydrates 4.2g	**1%**
Dietary Fiber 0.6g	**2%**
Sugars 2.5g	
Protein 43.5g	

Vitamin A 6%	•	Vitamin C 4%
Calcium 9%	•	Iron 79%

Nutrition Grade B
* Based on a 2000 calorie diet

Ingredients

- 5 cups Turkey, cooked and chopped
- 1 cup fresh Celery, finely chopped
- 1 fresh Jalapeno pepper, diced
- 3 tablespoons Dill Pickle Relish
- 1/2 cup Low-fat Sour cream
- 1/2 cup Low-fat Yogurt
- 1 tablespoon fresh Cilantro, chopped
- 1 teaspoons Black Pepper, ground
- 1/2 teaspoon Onion powder
- 1/2 teaspoon Garlic powder

Directions

1. **Combine** cooked turkey, celery, jalapeno, relish, sour cream and yogurt.

2. **Season** with cilantro, pepper, onion powder and garlic powder.
3. **Cover** and let chill until serving.

13. Hearty Corn Salad

Servings: 5

Preparation time: 10 minutes

Cook time: 10 minutes

Ready in: 20 minutes

Nutrition Facts

Serving Size 215 g

Amount Per Serving

Calories 163	Calories from Fat 35

% Daily Value*

Total Fat 3.9g	**6%**
Saturated Fat 0.7g	**4%**
Cholesterol 1mg	**0%**
Sodium 20mg	**1%**
Total Carbohydrates 29.4g	**10%**
Dietary Fiber 5.1g	**20%**
Sugars 9.7g	
Protein 5.8g	

Vitamin A 33%	•	Vitamin C 124%
Calcium 6%	•	Iron 15%

Nutrition Grade A

* Based on a 2000 calorie diet

Ingredients

- 1 tablespoon Olive Oil
- 2 cups Whole Kernel Corn, cooked
- 1/4 cup Black Beans, drained
- 1 Red Bell Pepper, sliced
- 1 Green Bell Pepper, sliced
- 1 cup chopped Zucchini
- 2 Green Onions, chopped
- 1 fresh Jalapeno Pepper, minced
- 4 Oz Cherry Tomato, halved, seeded
- 1 Lime, juiced
- 1/2 teaspoon Garlic powder
- 1/2 teaspoon Onion powder

- 1/2 cup Low-fat Greek Yogurt
- 2 tablespoons chopped fresh Coriander
- 1/2 teaspoon Black Pepper, ground

Directions

1. **Heat** oil in heavy large pan over medium-high heat. Stir in the corn, black beans, bell peppers, zucchini, green onions, jalapeno pepper, and tomato.
2. **Sauté** until vegetables are softened, or about 6 minutes. Remove from heat and refrigerate vegetables.
3. **Mix** lime juice, garlic and onion powder, and yogurt in a bowl. Add yogurt mixture into the vegetable mixture. Garnish with fresh chopped cilantro. Season with pepper to taste.

14. Fresh Garden Quinoa Vegetable Salad

Servings: 8

Preparation time: 20 minutes

Cook time: 25 minutes

Ready in: 45 minutes

Nutrition Facts

Serving Size 255 g

Amount Per Serving

Calories 231	Calories from Fat 61

	% Daily Value*
Total Fat 6.8g	**10%**
Saturated Fat 0.9g	**4%**
Trans Fat 0.0g	
Cholesterol 0mg	**0%**
Sodium 35mg	**1%**
Total Carbohydrates 34.7g	**12%**
Dietary Fiber 4.8g	**19%**
Sugars 2.9g	
Protein 7.5g	

Vitamin A 64%	•	Vitamin C 100%
Calcium 4%	•	Iron 15%

Nutrition Grade B+

* Based on a 2000 calorie diet

Ingredients

- 1 teaspoon Olive Oil
- 4 cloves Garlic, minced
- 1/4 cup Yellow Onion, diced
- 2 1/2 cups Low Sodium Chicken broth
- 1/4 teaspoon Black Pepper, ground
- 2 cups Quinoa
- 3/4 cup Cherry Tomato, diced
- 3/4 cup Carrots, shredded
- 1 Yellow Bell Pepper, diced
- 1 Red Bell Pepper, diced
- 1 Green Bell Pepper, diced
- 1 small Cucumber, diced

- 1/2 cup grilled Corn
- 1 1/2 tablespoons fresh Basil
- 1 tablespoon chopped fresh mint
- 1/4 teaspoon ground black pepper
- 2 tablespoons Olive Oil for drizzle
- 3 tablespoons White Wine

Directions

1. **Warm** the olive oil in a skillet over medium heat. Sauté garlic and 1/4 cup onion until the onion turned translucent or about 5 minutes. Pour in chicken broth and black pepper, and then bring to a boil.
2. **Add** the quinoa into the mixture. Reduce heat to medium-low, and simmer for about 20 minutes, or until the quinoa is tender.
3. **Remove** from heat and drain water from the quinoa with a strainer and transfer to a large mixing bowl. Refrigerate until chilled.
4. **Add** tomato, carrots, bell peppers, cucumber, and corn into the chilled quinoa. Season with basil, mint, and black pepper. Swirl with olive oil and white wine over the salad; mix well.

Snacks

Other than fast food, snack foods are probably the saltiest out there. Because they're often packaged, salt is used both as a flavor enhancer and a preservative, meaning that if you're not eating something that's fresh, you're almost certainly getting much more sodium than you bargained for. Even some of the snacks that I recommend, like pretzels, popcorn, and nuts, can be salty if you don't opt for low-salt versions, which can sometimes be hard to find if you're getting food while you're out.

Your best bet for snacks when you're out is produced—I know it's not always an option, but it's usually not too difficult to find some fresh fruit or vegetables that you can snack on. My personal strategy for this is to just keep a piece of fruit with me whenever I can and use it as an emergency snack to get me through an extra hour so I can find a healthy snack option.

Sticking with produce will help you avoid unhealthy fats as well—packaged snack foods, in addition to having a lot of salt, often contain trans fats, too. I hope it's becoming obvious why most snack foods are to be avoided! Fortunately, healthy snack foods are often high in fiber, so they won't leave you feeling hungry within half an hour.

Drinks

You might not think of drinks as having much salt in them, but you might be surprised to find out that there are actually a few that might contribute quite a bit to your daily sodium intake. For example, some blended coffee drinks can actually have over 200 mg of sodium in a serving! Be sure to check out the nutrition facts for drinks whenever you get the chance. Even some things like vegetable juice can have a surprising amount of salt (V8 is one that shows up on a lot of high-salt food lists). Oh, and to state the obvious, skip the salt on your margarita.

Fortunately, there aren't many drinks that include unhealthy fats. Or any fats, for that matter. As long as you don't have a cocktail that includes partially hydrogenated corn oil (and ask for skim milk in your coffee), you'll probably be okay.

Dinner

As you can see, any meal that you eat while you're out has the potential to have a lot of sodium—but I find dinner to be the hardest one to deal with. Dinner portions are often quite large, and the foods that are common at dinner are more likely to include rich sauces and condiments, as well as side dishes that can catch you off guard. It's hard to offer specific food recommendations for dinner, because of the wide variety of the things that you'll come across.

The best advice that I can offer is to use general strategies for limiting your sodium intake—ask for sauces and dressings on the side, so you can portion them yourself; avoid foods that have been pickled, smoked, or cured; avoid soy sauce and broth; skip salty appetizers in favor of fruits and vegetables. These are the kinds of tactics that will help you keep your sodium intake under control.

Because they're often so rich, dinner foods can be quite in high fat as well. A lot of the same strategies apply here—go really light on the sauces, choose foods that have been prepared using healthy methods, and skip the appetizers. You can also trim fat off of portions of your meat and ask that your vegetables be steamed and served without butter.

Of course, you won't always be able to make these changes to meals that you don't prepare yourself. Sometimes, you just won't have a choice. And in this case, I have a piece of advice for you: enjoy it. Don't stress over it, don't get down on yourself for having a high-sodium or high-fat meal. No one sticks to their diet 100% of the time.

So just enjoy a rich, delicious meal, and get back on the plan the next day!

1. Crispy Baked Cod

Servings: 4

Preparation time: 10 minutes

Cook time: 15 minutes

Ready in: 25 minutes

Nutrition Facts

Serving Size 230 g

Amount Per Serving

Calories 329	Calories from Fat 130

	% Daily Value*
Total Fat 14.5g	**22%**
Saturated Fat 3.8g	**19%**
Trans Fat 0.0g	
Cholesterol 53mg	**18%**
Sodium 270mg	**11%**
Total Carbohydrates 22.6g	**8%**
Dietary Fiber 1.2g	**5%**
Sugars 2.9g	
Protein 28.7g	

Vitamin A 4%	•	Vitamin C 8%
Calcium 19%	•	Iron 3%

Nutrition Grade C-

* Based on a 2000 calorie diet

Ingredients

- 3/4 cup Low-fat Milk
- 1/2 teaspoon Garlic powder
- 1/2 teaspoon Onion powder
- 3/4 cup Panko Original
- 1/4 cup grated Low-fat Parmesan cheese
- 1/4 teaspoon ground dried thyme
- 4 (4 Oz) Cod fillets
- 1 Lime, juiced
- 3 tablespoon Olive Oil
- 1 teaspoon Black Pepper, crushed

Directions

1. **Preheat** oven to 500 degrees F (260 degrees C).
2. **Mix** milk, lime juice, garlic powder and onion powder in a bowl. In a separate bowl, combine bread crumbs, Parmesan cheese, and thyme.
3. **Dip** the Cod fillets into the milk batter, then press into the crumb mixture and coat. Lay Cod fillets in a glass baking dish. Drizzle with oil and season with dash of pepper.
4. **Put** the dish on the top rack of the preheated oven and bake for 15 minutes.

2. Tilapia in Caper Cream Sauce

Servings: 4

Preparation time: 5 minutes

Cook time: 15 minutes

Ready in: 20 minutes

Nutrition Facts

Serving Size 146 g

Amount Per Serving

Calories 162   Calories from Fat 71

	% Daily Value*
Total Fat 7.9g	**12%**
Saturated Fat 1.4g	**7%**
Trans Fat 0.0g	
Cholesterol 46mg	**15%**
Sodium 189mg	**8%**
Total Carbohydrates 6.1g	**2%**
Dietary Fiber 0.9g	**4%**
Sugars 2.6g	
Protein 17.5g	

Vitamin A 3%   •   Vitamin C 14%
Calcium 7%   •   Iron 9%

Nutrition Grade C
* Based on a 2000 calorie diet

Ingredients

- 1 Lemon, juiced
- 1 teaspoon ground Black Pepper
- 1/2 teaspoon Thyme
- 1 tablespoon fresh Basil, chopped
- 1 teaspoon dried Dill Weed
- 1 teaspoon Garlic powder
- 2 (6 Oz) Tilapia fillets
- 2 tablespoons Olive Oil
- 1/2 cup Fat-free Half and Half
- 1 tablespoon Flour
- 2 tablespoons Capers, drained and rinsed

Directions

1. **Blend** lemon juice, pepper, thyme, basil, dill weed, and garlic powder in a small bowl. Rub mixture into the tilapia fillet. Set aside.

2. **Melt** butter in a large frying pan over medium heat. Lay fish in skillet, and increase heat to medium-high. Turn fillets frequently for about 5 minutes, or until lightly browned on both sides.

3. **Reduce** heat to medium. Cook 5 to 7 minutes more, until fillets are flaky. Remove fish fillets and transfer into a serving platter; cover with aluminum foil.

4. **Reheat** pan over high heat. Whisk half and half for about 3 minutes in the pan. Remove from heat. Stir in capers. Add flour if sauce is not thickened. Pour sauce over fish, and serve.

3. Cheese, Herbs & Spinach Stuffed Chicken Rolls

Servings: 2

Preparation time: 25 minutes

Cook time: 1 hour

Ready in: 1 hour and 25 minutes

Nutrition Facts

Serving Size 421 g

Amount Per Serving

Calories 339	Calories from Fat 87

	% Daily Value*
Total Fat 9.6g	**15%**
Saturated Fat 2.7g	**14%**
Trans Fat 0.0g	
Cholesterol 104mg	**35%**
Sodium 290mg	**12%**
Total Carbohydrates 21.5g	**7%**
Dietary Fiber 5.9g	**23%**
Sugars 9.1g	
Protein 43.3g	

Vitamin A 268%	•	Vitamin C 105%
Calcium 32%	•	Iron 35%

Nutrition Grade A

* Based on a 2000 calorie diet

Ingredients

- 1/2 cup Fat-free Yogurt
- 10 Oz fresh Spinach
- 1/4 cup 2% Low-fat Cottage Cheese with Sea Salt
- 2 cloves Garlic, chopped
- 1 Onion, chopped
- 2 (4 Oz) Chicken breasts, boneless & skinless
- 1 Lemon, juiced
- 1 teaspoon Black Pepper, crushed
- 1 teaspoon Garlic powder
- 1/2 teaspoon Thyme
- 1 teaspoon Rosemary

Directions

1. **Preheat** oven to 375 degrees F (190 degrees C).
2. **Combine** yogurt, spinach, cheese, onion and garlic. Mix well and set aside.
3. **Cut** small slit in each chicken breast enough for a spoonful of the spinach mixture to fit. Secure chicken breast with a toothpick and place in a baking dish.
4. **Drizzle** with lemon juice and season with pepper, garlic powder, thyme and rosemary; cover with foil.
5. **Bake** for 1 hour, or until the chicken juices run clear or internal temperature reaches 165 degrees F (74 degrees C).

4. Cous Cous topped with Asparagus Chicken Stir-fry

Servings: 4

Preparation time: 20 minutes

Cook time: 20 minutes

Ready in: 40 minutes

Nutrition Facts

Serving Size 356 g

Amount Per Serving

Calories 357	Calories from Fat 144

	% Daily Value*
Total Fat 16.0g	**25%**
Saturated Fat 2.1g	**11%**
Trans Fat 0.0g	
Cholesterol 24mg	**8%**
Sodium 122mg	**5%**
Total Carbohydrates 38.8g	**13%**
Dietary Fiber 4.0g	**16%**
Sugars 9.1g	
Protein 14.8g	

Vitamin A 46%	•	Vitamin C 138%
Calcium 3%	•	Iron 13%

Nutrition Grade B+

* Based on a 2000 calorie diet

Ingredients

- 1/2 pound fresh Asparagus, cut woody ends
- 3 tablespoons Coconut aminos
- 1 tablespoon Peanut Oil
- 1 tablespoon Raw honey
- 3 tablespoons Olive oil, divided
- 1 (4 Oz) Chicken breast, skinless, boneless, & cubed
- 2 cloves Garlic, minced
- ½ cup Mushroom, chopped
- 1 Green Bell Pepper, chopped
- 1 Red Bell Pepper, chopped
- 1 Red onion, minced

- 1 teaspoon Black Pepper, ground
- 2 cups Cous Cous

Directions

1. **Mix** together the asparagus, coconut aminos, peanut oil and honey and set aside. Cook cous cous, set aside and keep warm.
2. **Warm** 1 tablespoon of olive oil in a wok over medium high heat. Stir fry asparagus for about 2 minutes. Remove and set aside.
3. **Heat** the remaining olive oil in the same wok over high heat. Add chicken and stir fry until the chicken is no longer pink.
4. **Stir** in onion and garlic; cook until onion is softened. Toss in mushrooms, bell peppers, and reserved asparagus. Sprinkle with dash of black pepper. Serve over the hot Cous Cous.

5. Sweet and Spicy Chicken Kabobs

Servings: 12

Preparation time: 15 minutes

Cook time: 15 minutes

Ready in: 30 minutes

Nutrition Facts

Serving Size 169 g

Amount Per Serving

Calories 212	Calories from Fat 64

	% Daily Value*
Total Fat 7.1g	**11%**
Saturated Fat 0.6g	**3%**
Trans Fat 0.0g	
Cholesterol 65mg	**22%**
Sodium 326mg	**14%**
Total Carbohydrates 12.1g	**4%**
Dietary Fiber 1.7g	**7%**
Sugars 8.5g	
Protein 25.4g	

Vitamin A 20%	•	Vitamin C 73%
Calcium 2%	•	Iron 8%

Nutrition Grade A-

* Based on a 2000 calorie diet

Ingredients

- 1/4 cup Vegetable Oil, plus more for greasing
- 1/4 cup Raw Honey
- 1/3 cup Low Sodium Soy Sauce
- 1/4 teaspoon Black Pepper, ground
- 1/2 teaspoon Cayenne
- 1/2 teaspoon Chili
- ½ teaspoon sweet Paprika
- 1 tablespoon Rosemary, minced
- 1 Lemon, juiced
- 8 (4 Oz) skinless and boneless Chicken breast, cubed
- 2 cloves Garlic, crushed
- 5 small Onions, quartered

- 1 Red Bell Pepper, sliced
- 1 Green Bell Pepper, sliced
- 1 Yellow Bell Pepper, sliced
- 12 Cherry Tomato, halved

Directions

1. **Whisk** together the oil, honey, soy sauce, pepper, cayenne, chili, paprika, rosemary and lemon juice in a bowl, reserving ¼ of the marinade for later use. Add the chicken, garlic, onions, bell peppers and tomato in the bowl, and marinate in the refrigerator at least 2 hours.
2. **Preheat** the grill over high heat.
3. **Drain** liquid and discard from the chicken and vegetables. Insert chicken and vegetables alternately onto the skewers.
4. **Lightly brush** the grill grate with oil. Lay the skewers on the grill. Grill for 12 to 15 minutes, or until chicken juices run clear. Brush with the reserved marinade the both sides of the skewers, turning frequently.

6. Baked Chicken Breasts in Herb Basting Sauce

Servings: 4

Preparation time: 15 minutes

Cook time: 45 minutes

Ready in: 1 hour

Nutrition Facts

Serving Size 114 g

Amount Per Serving

Calories 204	Calories from Fat 114
	% Daily Value*
Total Fat 12.6g	**19%**
Saturated Fat 1.5g	**8%**
Trans Fat 0.0g	
Cholesterol 49mg	**16%**
Sodium 67mg	**3%**
Total Carbohydrates 5.0g	**2%**
Dietary Fiber 1.4g	**6%**
Sugars 1.6g	
Protein 18.9g	

Vitamin A 4%	•	Vitamin C 23%
Calcium 3%	•	Iron 8%

Nutrition Grade B+

* Based on a 2000 calorie diet

Ingredients

- 3 tablespoons Olive oil
- 1 Onion, minced
- 1 clove Garlic, crushed
- 1 teaspoon dried Thyme
- 1/2 teaspoon fresh Rosemary, minced
- 1/4 teaspoon fresh Sage, minced
- 1/4 teaspoon dried Marjoram
- 1/2 teaspoon Garlic powder
- 1/2 teaspoon Black Pepper, ground
- 1 Lemon, juiced
- 1/4 teaspoon Red Pepper flakes
- 4 boneless and skinless Chicken breast halves

- 1 teaspoon Lemon zest
- 1 1/2 tablespoons fresh Parsley, chopped

Directions

1. **Preheat** oven to 425 degrees F (220 degrees C).
2. **Combine** olive oil, onion, garlic, thyme, rosemary, sage, marjoram, garlic powder, pepper, lemon juice and red pepper flakes in a bowl.
3. **Dip** chicken breasts in sauce and coat all sides. Place skin side up in a shallow baking dish. Cover with foil.
4. **Roast** on preheated oven for about 35 to 45 minutes. Use pan drippings for basting. Remove and transfer into a warm platter, spoon pan juices and pour over the chicken. Sprinkle with lemon zest and fresh parsley.

7. Shrimp, Pineapple, Peppers Kabobs

Servings: 12

Preparation time: 25 minutes

Cook time: 5 minutes

Ready in: 30 minutes

Nutrition Facts

Serving Size 107 g

Amount Per Serving

Calories 92   Calories from Fat 28

	% Daily Value*
Total Fat 3.2g	**5%**
Saturated Fat 0.6g	**3%**
Cholesterol 80mg	**27%**
Sodium 101mg	**4%**
Total Carbohydrates 6.5g	**2%**
Dietary Fiber 1.4g	**5%**
Sugars 3.5g	
Protein 9.4g	

Vitamin A 28%   •   Vitamin C 100%

Calcium 5%   •   Iron 4%

Nutrition Grade A

* Based on a 2000 calorie diet

Ingredients

- 4 tablespoons Olive oil
- 1 Lemons, juiced
- 1 tablespoon Honey Mustard
- 1/2 cup fresh Basil leaves, minced
- 3 cloves Garlic, minced
- 1 teaspoon Onion powder
- 2 teaspoon White Pepper, ground
- 1 pound fresh Shrimp, peeled and deveined
- 1 cup Pineapple chunk
- 2 Red Bell Pepper, sliced
- 2 Green Bell Pepper, sliced
- 1 cup Mushroom, halved

Directions

1. **Mix** together olive oil, lemon juice, mustard, basil, and garlic, and season with onion powder and white pepper in a bowl. Toss in shrimp until coat. Cover with foil, and refrigerate for at least 1 hour.
2. **Preheat** grill over high heat. Remove shrimp from marinade. Thread shrimps alternately with pineapples, bell peppers and mushrooms.
3. **Brush** grill grate with oil, and arrange kabobs on the preheated grill. Cook for 4 minutes, turning once, or until smoky.

8. Teriyaki Pork and Vegetables Stir-fry

Servings: 4

Preparation time: 20 minutes

Cook time: 20 minutes

Ready in: 40 minutes

Nutrition Facts

Serving Size 322 g

Amount Per Serving

Calories 243	Calories from Fat 115

	% Daily Value*
Total Fat 12.8g	**20%**
Saturated Fat 2.9g	**14%**
Cholesterol 40mg	**13%**
Sodium 422mg	**18%**
Total Carbohydrates 17.6g	**6%**
Dietary Fiber 4.4g	**18%**
Sugars 6.6g	
Protein 16.9g	

Vitamin A 181%	•	Vitamin C 127%
Calcium 9%	•	Iron 18%

Nutrition Grade A-

* Based on a 2000 calorie diet

Ingredients

- 2 tablespoons Extra Virgin Olive oil
- 1/2 pound Pork Sirloin Chops, cubed
- 2 cloves Garlic, minced
- 2 tablespoons Low Sodium Soy Sauce
- 1 cup Broccoli, chopped
- 1 cup Green Bell Pepper, sliced
- 1 cup Baby Carrots
- 8 Oz Celery, sliced
- 1 cup fresh Bean Sprouts
- 1 cup Mushrooms, sliced
- 1 cup Green Onions, chopped
- 1 teaspoon Black Pepper, ground

- 1 teaspoon Onion powder
- 1/4 cup water
- 1/8 cup Pineapple juice
- 1/2 teaspoon Chili
- 1/2 teaspoon Black pepper
- 1 tablespoon flour

Directions

1. **Heat** oil in large heavy skillet over medium-high heat. Stir in pork, garlic and soy sauce, and sauté for 10 minutes.
2. **Toss** in broccoli, green pepper, carrots, celery, bean sprouts, mushrooms and green onions. Season with pepper and onion powder. Stir-fry for another 6 to 8 minutes.
3. **Whisk** together water, pineapple juice, chili, black pepper and flour. Pour mixture into vegetables, and cook until sauce is thickened.

9. Crispy Baked Fish & Chips

Servings: 4

Preparation time: 25 minutes

Cook time: 45 minutes

Ready in: 1 hour and 10 minutes

Nutrition Facts

Serving Size 382 g

Amount Per Serving

Calories 506	Calories from Fat 57

% Daily Value*

Total Fat 6.3g	**10%**
Saturated Fat 1.0g	**5%**
Trans Fat 0.0g	
Cholesterol 40mg	**13%**
Sodium 529mg	**22%**
Total Carbohydrates 76.3g	**25%**
Dietary Fiber 8.4g	**33%**
Sugars 5.9g	
Protein 35.0g	

Vitamin A 3%	•	Vitamin C 57%
Calcium 13%	•	Iron 22%

Nutrition Grade B+

* Based on a 2000 calorie diet

Ingredients

- 1 1/2 pound Potatoes
- 2 teaspoons Olive oil
- 1 teaspoon ground Fennel seed
- 1/2 teaspoon Paprika
- 1/2 teaspoon Cumin
- 1 teaspoon chopped fresh Coriander
- 1 teaspoon ground Black Pepper
- 2 cups Panko
- 1/4 cup Wholemeal flour
- 1 teaspoon Garlic powder
- 1 teaspoon Onion powder
- 3 egg whites

- 1 pound Cod fillet, cut into 4

Directions
1. **Preheat** oven to 425 degrees F (220 degrees C). Place racks in upper and lower rack of the oven. Brush a large baking sheet with little oil. Brush another cooking sheet with oil and set a wire rack on the sheet.
2. **Peel** potatoes and cut into wedges. Place into a colander and then rinse with cold water. Pat dry with paper towels. Transfer into shallow dish. Toss the potatoes, 1 tablespoon oil, fennel, paprika, cumin coriander, and pepper. Scatter onto the baking sheet without the rack. Place on the lower oven rack. Bake for 30 minutes, or until golden brown; turning every 10 minutes.
3. **Beat** egg white with pepper, garlic and onion powder. Add the remaining olive oil into Panko, mix well and set aside. Dust fish with the flour, dip into egg batter, and coat all side with Panko. Place on the prepared wire rack.
4. **Place** the fish on the upper oven rack. Bake for 20 minutes, or until opaque in the center and crispy on the outside.

10. Chicken Thighs in Raspberry Vinegar Sauce

Servings: 4

Preparation time: 10 minutes

Cook time: 25 minutes

Ready in: 35 minutes

Nutrition Facts

Serving Size 192 g

Amount Per Serving

Calories 341   Calories from Fat 185

% Daily Value*

Total Fat 20.5g	**32%**
Saturated Fat 5.4g	**27%**
Trans Fat 0.0g	
Cholesterol 107mg	**36%**
Sodium 112mg	**5%**
Total Carbohydrates 3.4g	**1%**
Dietary Fiber 0.9g	**4%**
Sugars 0.7g	
Protein 34.1g	

Vitamin A 3%   •   Vitamin C 3%

Calcium 5%   •   Iron 14%

Nutrition Grade C+

* Based on a 2000 calorie diet

Ingredients

- 3 tablespoon Vegetable oil
- 4 (4 Oz) bone-in Chicken Thighs, skinless
- 3 tablespoons Red Onion, minced
- 1 teaspoon fresh Rosemary
- 1 teaspoon fresh Thyme
- 1 teaspoon fresh Marjoram
- 1 teaspoon dried Oregano
- 1/2 cup Mushrooms, sliced
- 1/3 cup Low Sodium Chicken stock
- 1/4 cup Raspberry Vinegar
- 1/4 cup Half and Half
- 1 teaspoon Garlic powder

- 1 teaspoon Black Pepper, ground

Directions

1. **Heat** oil in a large skillet over medium heat. Stir in the chicken and cook until browned on both sides or until the juices run clear. Remove from pan and set aside.
2. **Sauté** the onion, rosemary, thyme, marjoram, oregano, and mushrooms on the pan. Pour chicken stock and simmer for 3 minutes.
3. **Add** the raspberry vinegar. Bring to a boil, stirring occasionally, until the mixture thickens. Stir in the half and half, and then return the chicken to the skillet. Cook for a minute, turning the chicken pieces to coat well with the sauce. Season with garlic powder and pepper to taste.

11. 3 Cheese Veggie Lasagna

Servings: 12

Preparation time: 25 minutes

Cook time: 1 hour

Ready in: 1 hour and 25 minutes

Nutrition Facts

Serving Size 250 g

Amount Per Serving

Calories 334	Calories from Fat 116

% Daily Value*

Total Fat 12.9g	**20%**
Saturated Fat 5.5g	**28%**
Trans Fat 0.0g	
Cholesterol 37mg	**12%**
Sodium 563mg	**23%**
Total Carbohydrates 38.9g	**13%**
Dietary Fiber 3.5g	**14%**
Sugars 9.7g	
Protein 17.4g	

Vitamin A 45%	•	Vitamin C 53%
Calcium 30%	•	Iron 5%

Nutrition Grade B-

* Based on a 2000 calorie diet

Ingredients

- 16 Oz Lasagna noodles
- 8 Oz fresh Portabella Mushrooms, sliced
- 1 Green Bell Pepper, chopped
- 1 Red Bell Pepper, chopped
- 1 Carrot, shredded
- 1 Zucchini, chopped
- 1 large Onion, chopped
- 3 cloves Garlic, minced
- 2 tablespoons Olive oil
- 1 teaspoon fresh basil, chopped
- 4 cups Pasta Sauce
- 8 Oz Low-fat Ricotta cheese

- 8 Oz Low- fat Mozzarella cheese
- 2 egg whites
- 4 Oz grated Low-fat Parmesan cheese

Directions

1. **Preheat** oven to 350 degrees F (175 degrees C).
2. **Fill** half of the large pot with water and bring to boil. Cook lasagna noodles until al dente. Rinse with cold water, and drain.
3. **Heat** olive oil in a saucepan over medium- high heat. Cook mushrooms, bell peppers, carrot, zucchini, onion, and garlic. Pour in pasta sauce and add basil; bring to a boil. Reduce the heat, and simmer 15 minutes.
4. **Whisk** together ricotta, half of the mozzarella cheese, and eggs.
5. **Grease** a 9x13 inch baking dish. Cover the bottom with 1 cup pasta sauce. Layer 1/2 each, lasagna noodles, ricotta mix, pasta sauce, and Parmesan cheese. Repeat the layering until all lasagna noodles is used. Top with remaining of the mozzarella cheese. Uncovered.
6. **Bake** on preheated oven for 40 minutes. Remove from oven and let stand for about 15 minutes before serving.

12. Simple Everyday Ratatouille

Servings: 8

Preparation time: 10 minutes

Cook time: 30 minutes

Ready in: 40 minutes

Nutrition Facts

Serving Size 229 g

Amount Per Serving

Calories 169	Calories from Fat 119

	% Daily Value*
Total Fat 13.2g	**20%**
Saturated Fat 1.9g	**9%**
Trans Fat 0.0g	
Cholesterol 0mg	**0%**
Sodium 12mg	**0%**
Total Carbohydrates 13.3g	**4%**
Dietary Fiber 5.2g	**21%**
Sugars 6.0g	
Protein 2.5g	

Vitamin A 33%	•	Vitamin C 132%
Calcium 5%	•	Iron 23%

Nutrition Grade A-

* Based on a 2000 calorie diet

Ingredients

- 1/2 cup olive oil
- 2 White Onion, sliced into rings
- 3 cloves Garlic, crushed then minced
- 1 Zucchini, cubed
- 1 Eggplant, cubed
- 1 Yellow Squash, cubed
- 1 Green Bell Peppers, chopped
- 1 Red Bell Pepper, chopped
- 1 Yellow Bell Pepper, chopped
- 2 Beefsteak tomatoes, sliced
- 1 Bay leaf
- 4 sprigs fresh thyme

- 1 tablespoon Balsamic Vinegar
- 1 teaspoon Black Pepper, ground
- 2 tablespoons fresh Parsley, chopped

Directions

1. **Heat** 1 1/2 tablespoon of the olive oil in a large pot over medium-low heat. Sauté the onions and garlic until softened.
2. **Sauté** the zucchini in 1 ½ olive oil, on a separate skillet over medium heat. Cook until slightly browned on all sides. Remove the zucchini and transfer in the pot with the onions and garlic.
3. **Reheat** skillet and add 1 ½ of olive oil over medium heat. Cook all remaining vegetables. Remove from skillet and then transfer into the pot.
4. **Season** vegetables in the pot with balsamic vinegar and pepper. Add the bay leaf and thyme and cover with lid. Cook for 20 minutes over medium heat.
5. **Toss** in chopped tomatoes and parsley into the pot; cook for another 10-15 minutes. Stirring occasionally.
6. **Remove** the bay leaf and serve warm.

13. Spicy Vegetable and Beef Soup

Servings: 8

Preparation time: 10 minutes

Cook time: 50 minutes

Ready in: 1 hour

Nutrition Facts

Serving Size 336 g

Amount Per Serving

Calories 181 | Calories from Fat 38

	% Daily Value*
Total Fat 4.2g	6%
Saturated Fat 1.5g	7%
Cholesterol 51mg	17%
Sodium 271mg	11%
Total Carbohydrates 14.4g	5%
Dietary Fiber 4.2g	17%
Sugars 6.4g	
Protein 21.7g	

Vitamin A 50% • Vitamin C 101%
Calcium 4% • Iron 67%

Nutrition Grade A
* Based on a 2000 calorie diet

Ingredients

- 1 pound ground Beef
- 2 cups Low Sodium Beef broth
- 2 cups Low Sodium Tomato Juice
- 8 Oz Cherry Tomato, halved
- 1 White Onion, chopped
- 1 cup Broccoli, chopped
- 1 cup Cauliflower, chopped
- 4 Oz Baby Carrot
- 1/2 cup Green Peas
- 1/2 cup Corn
- 1 teaspoon ground black pepper
- 1 teaspoon Garlic powder

- 1 teaspoon Cayenne
- 1/2 teaspoon Red Pepper flakes

Directions

1. **Cook** ground beef in a large pot over medium heat, until browned. Drain.
2. **Pour** in beef broth and tomato juice. Add tomatoes, onion, broccoli, cauliflower, carrots, peas, corn, pepper, garlic powder, cayenne and pepper flakes into the pot. Bring to a boil.
3. **Reduce** the heat and simmer about 45 minutes.
4. **Serve** warm.

14. Pork Vegetable Tomato Soup

Servings: 8

Preparation time: 10 minutes

Cook time: 30 minutes

Ready in: 40 minutes

Nutrition Facts

Serving Size 271 g

Amount Per Serving

Calories 210	Calories from Fat 85

% Daily Value*

Total Fat 9.4g	**15%**
Saturated Fat 3.8g	**19%**
Trans Fat 0.0g	
Cholesterol 53mg	**18%**
Sodium 220mg	**9%**
Total Carbohydrates 10.4g	**3%**
Dietary Fiber 3.2g	**13%**
Sugars 4.7g	
Protein 21.8g	

Vitamin A 24%	•	Vitamin C 94%
Calcium 10%	•	Iron 14%

Nutrition Grade A

* Based on a 2000 calorie diet

Ingredients

- 2 teaspoons Olive oil
- 1 pound Lean Pork, cubed
- 1 Yellow Onion, chopped
- 3 cloves Garlic, minced
- 1 Red Bell Pepper, chopped
- 1 Green Bell Pepper, chopped
- 2 Zucchini, quartered and sliced
- ½ cup Tomato Sauce
- 8 Oz fresh Mushrooms, sliced
- 1 cup Tomato, diced
- 1 Artichoke, quartered
- 1 cup Low Sodium Chicken broth

- 1/2 cup Cream
- 2 teaspoons fresh Basil, chopped
- 1 teaspoon dried Oregano
- 1 teaspoon Black Pepper, ground
- 2 Oz grated Low-fat Parmesan cheese

Directions

1. **Heat** 1 teaspoon olive oil in a skillet over medium high heat. Stir in pork and cook for about 8 to 10 minutes or until browned on all sides. Set aside.
2. **Warm** remaining of the olive oil in an 8 quart saucepan over medium heat. Stir in the onions, garlic and bell pepper. Sauté for just a few minutes until softened.
3. **Add** the cooked pork, zucchini, tomato sauce, mushrooms, diced tomatoes, artichoke, chicken broth, cream, basil, oregano, black pepper. Cover and simmer for 20 minutes. Sprinkle with cheese and serve.

DESSERT

1. Nutty Caramel Apples

Servings: 6

Preparation time: 8 minutes

Cook time: 2 minutes

Ready in: 10 minutes

Nutrition Facts

Serving Size 272 g

Amount Per Serving

Calories 488   Calories from Fat 262

	% Daily Value*
Total Fat 29.1g	**45%**
Saturated Fat 13.8g	**69%**
Trans Fat 0.0g	
Cholesterol 0mg	**0%**
Sodium 59mg	**2%**
Total Carbohydrates 67.5g	**22%**
Dietary Fiber 6.2g	**25%**
Sugars 20.0g	
Protein 7.5g	

Vitamin A 3%	•	Vitamin C 15%
Calcium 4%	•	Iron 5%

Nutrition Grade C-

* Based on a 2000 calorie diet

Ingredients
- 6 apples, stem removed
- 14 Oz Caramel pack
- 2 tablespoons Low-fat Milk
- 1/4 cup Pistachios, finely chopped
- 1/4 cup Walnuts, finely chopped
- 1/4 cup Almond, finely chopped
- 1/4 cup Pecans, finely chopped

Directions
1. **Press** a craft stick into the top of each apple.

2. **Place** in a microwavable bowl the caramel and milk. Microwave for 2 minutes, stirring once. Let cool for a minute.
3. **Roll** each apple into the caramel sauce and then into the mixed nuts bed, coat well and serve.

2. Carrot Cake with Almonds

Servings: 15

Preparation time: 20 minutes

Cook time: 1hour

Ready in: 1 hour and 20 minutes

Nutrition Facts

Serving Size 111 g

Amount Per Serving

Calories 281   Calories from Fat 106

% **Daily Value***

Total Fat 11.8g   **18%**

Saturated Fat 3.3g   **17%**

Trans Fat 0.0g

Cholesterol 42mg   **14%**

Sodium 257mg   **11%**

Total Carbohydrates 39.1g   **13%**

Dietary Fiber 3.1g   **12%**

Sugars 19.5g

Protein 6.2g

Vitamin A 63%   •   Vitamin C 4%

Calcium 6%   •   Iron 14%

Nutrition Grade C-

* Based on a 2000 calorie diet

Ingredients

- 2 cups all-purpose flour, plus more for dusting pan
- 2 teaspoons baking soda
- 1 1/2 cups sugar
- 1 teaspoon ground cinnamon
- 3/4 cup low-fat buttermilk
- 1/4 cup olive oil, plus more for greasing pan
- 2 cups carrots, shredded
- 3 eggs, beaten
- 1 cup flaked coconut
- 1 cup almonds, chopped
- 1 cup dried cranberries (or raisins)
- 2 teaspoons vanilla extract

Directions

1. **Preheat** oven to 350 degrees F (175 degrees C). Grease and flour an 8x12 inch pan.
2. **Sift** together the baking soda, flour, cinnamon, and sugar in a medium bowl. Set aside.
3. **Combine** the buttermilk, eggs, oil, and vanilla in a large bowl. Mix in the flour mixture. Fold in the coconut, carrots, raisins and almonds. Pour batter into the prepared pan.
4. **Bake** for 1 hour. Insert a toothpick into the center of the cake. The cake is cooked if the toothpick comes out clean or with only a few crumbs sticking to it. Let cool before serving.

3. Egg white Crepes

Servings: 8

Preparation time: 10 minutes

Cook time: 10 minutes

Ready in: 20 minutes

Nutrition Facts

Serving Size 96 g

Amount Per Serving

Calories 99	Calories from Fat 45

	% Daily Value*
Total Fat 5.0g	**8%**
Saturated Fat 2.1g	**11%**
Trans Fat 0.0g	
Cholesterol 10mg	**3%**
Sodium 74mg	**3%**
Total Carbohydrates 7.7g	**3%**
Dietary Fiber 0.5g	**2%**
Sugars 6.9g	
Protein 5.8g	

Vitamin A 3%	•	Vitamin C 0%
Calcium 6%	•	Iron 1%

Nutrition Grade C-

* Based on a 2000 calorie diet

Ingredients

- 8 egg white, lightly beaten
- 1 1/3 cups Low-fat Milk
- 2 tablespoons Unsalted Danish Butter, melted
- 1 cup Almond flour
- 2 tablespoons Raw Honey
- 1 teaspoon Vanilla Extract
- 1 teaspoon ground Cinnamon

Directions

1. **Whisk** together egg white, milk, melted butter, flour, honey, vanilla extract and cinnamon until evenly smooth.

2. **Heat** a medium-sized frying pan over medium heat. Grease pan. Scope 3 tablespoons crepe batter into hot pan, tilt pan to coat the bottom surface. Cook over medium heat, for 1 to 2 minutes on each side, or until golden brown.

3. **Serve** warm.

4. Easy Berry Cobbler

Servings: 4

Preparation time: 10 minutes

Cook time: 1 hour

Ready in: 1 hour and 10 minutes

Nutrition Facts

Serving Size 173 g

Amount Per Serving

Calories 274   Calories from Fat 129

	% Daily Value*
Total Fat 14.3g	**22%**
Saturated Fat 7.5g	**38%**
Trans Fat 0.0g	
Cholesterol 32mg	**11%**
Sodium 23mg	**1%**
Total Carbohydrates 33.5g	**11%**
Dietary Fiber 3.9g	**16%**
Sugars 27.9g	
Protein 3.3g	

Vitamin A 8%   •   Vitamin C 31%
Calcium 13%   •   Iron 3%

Nutrition Grade C+

* Based on a 2000 calorie diet

Ingredients

- 4 tablespoons Unsalted Danish Butter
- 3/4 cup Almond flour
- 1/3 cup Organic Agave Nectar
- 1 teaspoon Baking powder
- 3/4 cup Low-fat Milk
- 1/2 cup fresh Strawberry
- 1/2 cup fresh Blueberry
- 1/2 cup fresh Raspberry
- 1/2 cup fresh Cherry

Directions

1. **Preheat** oven to 350 degrees F (180 degrees C). Arrange oven rack to upper-middle position.
2. **Place** butter in a 9-inch round pan; place into the oven to melt. Remove from oven.
3. **Whisk** flour, agave, and baking powder in small bowl. Add the milk; whisk to form a soft batter. Pour batter into the round pan. Scatter the berries over the batter.
4. **Bake** for 50 minutes or until batter browns. Serve warm a scoop of vanilla ice cream, if desired.

* When baking with agave, honey, or molasses, lowers the oven temperature by 25 degrees to avoid overbrowning.

5. Cinnamon Crumb Banana Muffins

Servings: 6

Preparation time: 15 minutes

Cook time: 18 minutes

Ready in: 35 Minutes

Nutrition Facts

Serving Size 68 g

Amount Per Serving

Calories 178   Calories from Fat 43

% Daily Value*

	% Daily Value*
Total Fat 4.8g	**7%**
Saturated Fat 2.6g	**13%**
Trans Fat 0.0g	
Cholesterol 27mg	**9%**
Sodium 254mg	**11%**
Total Carbohydrates 30.6g	**10%**
Dietary Fiber 1.0g	**4%**
Sugars 14.8g	
Protein 3.6g	

Vitamin A 1%	•	Vitamin C 3%
Calcium 4%	•	Iron 6%

Nutrition Grade C-

* Based on a 2000 calorie diet

Ingredients
- 3/4 cup and 1 1/2 tablespoons all-purpose flour, divided
- 1/2 teaspoon baking soda
- 1/2 teaspoon baking powder
- 1/4 teaspoon salt
- 1/3 cup and 3 tablespoons brown sugar, divided
- 4 tablespoons melted low-fat butter
- 1 egg
- 1-3/4 banana, mashed
- 1/8 teaspoon ground cinnamon
- 1/2 teaspoon vanilla extract

Directions

1. **Preheat** oven to 375 degrees F (190 degrees C). Line 6 muffin cups with muffin papers.
2. **Mix** together the 3/4 cup flour, baking powder, baking soda, and salt in a large bowl. In another bowl, beat together the 1/3 cup sugar, 3 tablespoons butter and egg. Fold in the mashed banana and combine thoroughly; stirring just until moistened. Divide the batter among the prepared muffin cups.
3. **Stir** together the cinnamon, vanilla, and remaining sugar and flour in a small bowl. Mix in the remaining 1 tablespoons butter until the mixture becomes coarse. Sprinkle topping over muffins.
4. **Bake** for 18 to 20 minutes. Insert a toothpick into the center of each muffin; if it comes out clean it's done, else return the muffins to the oven and bake for a few more minutes.

6. Protein-Rich Pumpkin Cookies

Servings: 7

Preparation time: 15 minutes

Cook time: 5-10 minutes

Ready in: 20 minutes

Nutrition Facts

Serving Size 100 g

Amount Per Serving

Calories 139   Calories from Fat 35

         % Daily Value*

Total Fat 3.9g	**6%**
Trans Fat 0.0g	
Cholesterol 0mg	**0%**
Sodium 402mg	**17%**
Total Carbohydrates 25.2g	**8%**
Dietary Fiber 3.3g	**13%**
Sugars 11.7g	
Protein 3.3g	

Vitamin A 109%   •   Vitamin C 3%

Calcium 5%   •   Iron 8%

Nutrition Grade B+

* Based on a 2000 calorie diet

Ingredients

- 1/4 cup raw honey
- 1 cup rolled oats
- 1 1/2 cup almond flour
- 1 3/4 teaspoons baking soda
- 1/2 teaspoon baking powder
- 1/4 teaspoon salt
- 2 teaspoons ground cinnamon
- 1 cup pumpkin puree
- 1 tablespoon applesauce
- 2 tablespoons cornstarch mixed with 6 tablespoons water
- 1/2 teaspoon allspice

Directions

1. **Preheat** oven to 350 degrees F (175 degrees C).
2. **Mix** together all the ingredients gradually in a large bowl. Shape batter into 12 balls and flatten on a baking sheet; arrange 2 inches apart.
3. **Bake** for 5 minutes.

7. Easy Banana Berry Parfait

Servings: 1

Preparation time: 10 minutes

Cook time: 10 minutes

Ready in: 20 minutes

Nutrition Facts

Serving Size 424 g

Amount Per Serving

Calories 459   Calories from Fat 103

% Daily Value*

	% Daily Value*
Total Fat 11.4g	**18%**
Saturated Fat 2.0g	**10%**
Trans Fat 0.0g	
Cholesterol 0mg	**0%**
Sodium 12mg	**1%**
Total Carbohydrates 73.5g	**24%**
Dietary Fiber 10.5g	**42%**
Sugars 34.2g	
Protein 19.0g	

Vitamin A 3%	•	Vitamin C 109%
Calcium 5%	•	Iron 17%

Nutrition Grade A

* Based on a 2000 calorie diet

Ingredients

- 1/2 cup fresh Strawberries, sliced
- 4 Oz Fat-free Greek yogurt
- 1/2 cup fresh Blueberries, sliced
- 1 banana, sliced
- 1 tablespoon Wheat Germ
- 1/3 cup Granola

Directions

1. **Layer** strawberries, 1/3 of yogurt, blueberries, 1/3 of the yogurt, banana slices, the remaining of the yogurt, granola and sprinkle of wheat germ in a glass dessert bowl.
2. **Chill** before serving.

8. Pecan and Cranberry Oatmeal Cookies

Servings: 12

Preparation time: 15 minutes

Cook time: 10 minutes

Ready in: 25 minutes

Nutrition Facts

Serving Size 72 g

Amount Per Serving

Calories 204   Calories from Fat 132

	% Daily Value*
Total Fat 14.6g	**23%**
Saturated Fat 5.3g	**27%**
Trans Fat 0.0g	
Cholesterol 20mg	**7%**
Sodium 179mg	**7%**
Total Carbohydrates 14.4g	**5%**
Dietary Fiber 2.6g	**10%**
Sugars 7.0g	
Protein 3.6g	

Vitamin A 4%   •   Vitamin C 4%
Calcium 2%   •   Iron 4%

Nutrition Grade D
* Based on a 2000 calorie diet

Ingredients

- 8 tablespoons Danish Butter
- 1/4 cup Raw Honey
- 4 egg whites
- 1 teaspoon vanilla extract
- 1/4 teaspoon Nutmeg
- 1 teaspoon Cinnamon
- 1 2/3 cups Almond flour
- 1 1/2 teaspoons Baking soda
- 1 cup Rolled Oats
- 3/4 cup Pecans, chopped
- 2 cups fresh Cranberries, chopped

Directions

1. **Preheat** oven to 350 degrees F (175 degrees C).
2. **Mix** butter and honey until smooth. Add egg whites, vanilla, cinnamon and nutmeg. Mix well.
3. **Sift** flour and baking soda together in a separate bowl. Whisk into butter mixture. Add in the rolled oats. Fold in nuts and cranberries. Scoop a spoonful of the dough onto ungreased cookie dish, leaving 2 inch apart.
4. **Bake** onto the preheated oven for 10 minutes, or until the edges are crusty and the centers are dry. Let sit on wire racks just before serving.

* When baking with agave, honey, or molasses, lower the oven temperature by 25 degrees to avoid overbrowning.

9. Easy Blackberry Pie

Servings: 8

Preparation time: 30 minutes

Cook time: 35 minutes

Ready in: 1 hour and 5 minutes

Nutrition Facts

Serving Size 138 g

Amount Per Serving

Calories 264	Calories from Fat 126

	% Daily Value*
Total Fat 14.1g	**22%**
Saturated Fat 3.3g	**16%**
Trans Fat 0.0g	
Cholesterol 7mg	**2%**
Sodium 156mg	**6%**
Total Carbohydrates 32.7g	**11%**
Dietary Fiber 5.3g	**21%**
Sugars 20.3g	
Protein 4.0g	

Vitamin A 8%	•	Vitamin C 24%
Calcium 5%	•	Iron 8%

Nutrition Grade C+

* Based on a 2000 calorie diet

Ingredients

- 9 inch Graham Crackers Pie Crust
- 1/4 cup Organic Agave Nectar
- 3 tablespoons Almond flour
- 1 tablespoon Lemon juice
- 2 tablespoons Danish Butter
- 1/2 teaspoon ground Cinnamon
- 4 cups fresh Blackberries, rinsed and drained

Directions

1. **Whisk** agave, tablespoons flour, lemon juice, butter and cinnamon in a large bowl. Mix until evenly smooth. Toss in the berries. Pour berry filling into the pie crust.
2. **Place** on the lower shelf of the oven in a 425 degree F (220 degree C). Bake for 30 minutes or until desired doneness.

* When baking with agave, honey, or molasses, lower the oven temperature by 25 degrees to avoid overbrowning.

10. Fruity Coconutty Salad

Servings: 12

Preparation time: 20 minutes

Nutrition Facts

Serving Size 206 g

Amount Per Serving

Calories 187	Calories from Fat 70

% Daily Value*

Total Fat 7.8g	**12%**
Saturated Fat 4.0g	**20%**
Trans Fat 0.0g	
Cholesterol 5mg	**2%**
Sodium 55mg	**2%**
Total Carbohydrates 25.0g	**8%**
Dietary Fiber 3.5g	**14%**
Sugars 20.2g	
Protein 5.4g	

Vitamin A 7%	•	Vitamin C 53%
Calcium 15%	•	Iron 10%

Nutrition Grade B+

* Based on a 2000 calorie diet

Ingredients

- 2 Mangoes, cubed
- 1 small Pineapple, chunked
- 2 Apples, chunked
- 1/2 cup Green grapes, halved
- 3 1/2 cups Low-fat Yogurt
- 1 1/2 cups shredded Coconut
- 1 cup Cherries
- 1/2 cup Fat-free Whipped Cream
- 1/2 cup toasted Pecans, chopped

Directions

1. **Toss** the mangoes, pineapple, apple, grapes, yogurt, coconut, cherries and whipped cream in a large glass bowl.
2. **Mix** well and refrigerate for 1 hour. Sprinkle some toasted pecans on top just before serving.

11. Zesty Cranberry Almond Biscotti

Servings: 7

Preparation time: 25 minutes

Cook time: 45 minutes

Ready in: 1 hour and 10 minutes

Nutrition Facts

Serving Size 106 g

Amount Per Serving

Calories 270	Calories from Fat 157

	% Daily Value*
Total Fat 17.5g	**27%**
Saturated Fat 1.8g	**9%**
Trans Fat 0.0g	
Cholesterol 0mg	**0%**
Sodium 35mg	**1%**
Total Carbohydrates 25.2g	**8%**
Dietary Fiber 3.1g	**12%**
Sugars 20.0g	
Protein 6.5g	

Vitamin A 0%	•	Vitamin C 4%
Calcium 8%	•	Iron 5%

Nutrition Grade D+

* Based on a 2000 calorie diet

Ingredients

- 1/4 cup light Olive oil
- 1/2 cup Organic Agave Nectar
- 3 teaspoon almond extract
- 1 teaspoon Orange juice
- 4 eggs white
- 1 3/4 cups Almond flour
- 1 teaspoon Baking powder
- 1 cup fresh Cranberries
- ½ teaspoon Orange zest
- 1 cup slivered Almond

Directions

1. **Preheat** oven to 300 degrees F (150 degrees C).
2. **Combine** together oil and agave in a large bowl until smooth. Mix in the almond extracts, orange juice, and then beat in the egg whites. Sift in flour and baking powder, slowly stirring onto mixture to avoid lumps. Toss in cranberries, orange zest and nuts. Make the dough by your clean hands.
3. **Make** two 12x12 inch logs out from the dough and lay them in a cookie sheet with parchment paper. Wet hands with cool water to handle the sticky dough easily.
4. **Bake** in the preheated oven for 35 minutes. Remove from oven and let sit for 10 minutes to cool. Decrease oven heat to 275 degrees F (135 degrees C).
5. **Slice** logs into 3/4 inch diagonal thick cuts. Arrange cookies on parchment covered cookie sheet. Bake for 10 minutes, or until center is dry. Let cool and serve.

* When baking with agave, honey, or molasses, lower the oven temperature by 25 degrees to avoid overbrowning.

12. Lower Fat Fudge Brownies

Servings: 9

Preparation time: 10 minutes

Cook time: 30 minutes

Ready in: 40 minutes

Nutrition Facts

Serving Size 70 g

Amount Per Serving

Calories 120	Calories from Fat 14

% Daily Value*

Total Fat 1.5g	**2%**
Saturated Fat 0.5g	**3%**
Trans Fat 0.0g	
Cholesterol 1mg	**0%**
Sodium 177mg	**7%**
Total Carbohydrates 25.7g	**9%**
Dietary Fiber 2.8g	**11%**
Sugars 21.4g	
Protein 3.7g	

Vitamin A 0%	Vitamin C 0%
Calcium 4%	Iron 4%

Nutrition Grade B

* Based on a 2000 calorie diet

Ingredients

- 3/4 cup Organic Agave Nectar
- 6 tablespoons unsweetened Cocoa powder
- 1 teaspoon Balsamic Vinegar
- 10 tablespoons Low-fat Vanilla Yogurt
- 1/2 teaspoon Cinnamon
- 4 egg whites
- 1/2 cup Almond flour
- 1 tablespoon all-purpose flour
- 1 teaspoon Baking Soda
- Coconut oil for greasing

Directions

1. **Preheat** oven to 325 degrees F (165 degrees C). Grease an 8x8 inch baking dish lightly with coconut oil.

2. **Mix** together the agave, cocoa powder, balsamic vinegar, and yogurt in a large bowl. Beat in the egg whites until smooth. Stir in the flours and baking soda until rapt. Pour batter into the prepared pan.

3. **Bake** in the preheated oven for 28 minutes, or until the toothpick inserted into the center comes out clean. Let the brownies to cool before cutting into squares and serving.

* When baking with agave, honey, or molasses, lower the oven temperature by 25 degrees to avoid overbrowning.

13. Minty Double Chocolate Cookies

Servings: 8

Preparation time: 8 minutes

Cook time: 10-11 minutes

Ready in: 18 minutes

Nutrition Facts

Serving Size 41 g

Amount Per Serving

Calories 192   Calories from Fat 126

	% Daily Value*
Total Fat 14.0g	**22%**
Saturated Fat 6.9g	**35%**
Trans Fat 0.0g	
Cholesterol 1mg	**0%**
Sodium 55mg	**2%**
Total Carbohydrates 14.2g	**5%**
Dietary Fiber 3.7g	**15%**
Sugars 7.6g	
Protein 5.0g	

Vitamin A 0%   •   Vitamin C 0%
Calcium 4%   •   Iron 23%

Nutrition Grade D+
* Based on a 2000 calorie diet

Ingredients

- 1 cup almond meal
- 1/8 teaspoon sea salt
- 1 cup pure cocoa powder
- 1/8 teaspoon baking soda
- 1/4 cup dark chocolate, chopped
- 3 tablespoons coconut oil, melted
- 2 tablespoons raw honey
- 1 tablespoon almond milk
- 1 tablespoon pure mint extract
- 1 teaspoon pure vanilla extract

Directions

1. **Preheat** oven to 350 degrees F. Line a baking sheet with parchment paper.
2. **Mix** together the almond meal, baking soda, cocoa powder, salt, and dark chocolate in a medium bowl. Whisk together coconut oil, honey, almond milk, mint extract, and vanilla in a small bowl.
3. **Pour** wet mixture over dry mixture and stir well to combine.
4. **Fill** a tablespoon or cookie scoop with batter and drop 2 inches apart out onto the prepared baking sheet. Lightly press down in the center.
5. **Bake** for 10-11 minutes, or until set. Remove from oven and let cool in a wire rack.
6. **Store** cookies in a tightly covered cookie jar.

14. Berry Nutty Bars

Servings: 10

Preparation time: 20 minutes

Cook time: 45 minutes

Ready in: 1 hour and 5 minutes

Nutrition Facts

Serving Size 80 g

Amount Per Serving

Calories 260   Calories from Fat 172

	% Daily Value*
Total Fat 19.1g	**29%**
Saturated Fat 8.8g	**44%**
Trans Fat 0.0g	
Cholesterol 36mg	**12%**
Sodium 3mg	**0%**
Total Carbohydrates 18.7g	**6%**
Dietary Fiber 1.5g	**6%**
Sugars 15.7g	
Protein 2.7g	

Vitamin A 8%	•	Vitamin C 17%
Calcium 2%	•	Iron 3%

Nutrition Grade C-

* Based on a 2000 calorie diet

Ingredients

- 1 1/2 cups Almond flour
- 1/2 cup Raw Honey
- 3/4 cup Danish Butter, softened
- 1/4 cup sliced fresh Raspberry
- 1/2 cup sliced fresh Strawberry
- 1/4 cup sliced fresh Blueberry
- 1/4 cup sliced fresh Blackberry
- 1/4 cup fresh Orange juice
- 1 tablespoon Cornstarch
- 1/2 cup Walnuts, chopped

Directions

1. **Preheat** oven to 350 degrees F (190 degrees C).
2. **Mix** the flour, honey and butter in the electric mixer. Place into a 13x9 inch ungreased baking pan. Bake on the preheated oven at 350 degrees F (175 degrees C) for 15 minutes.
3. **Place** the berries, orange juice, and cornstarch in a large saucepan over medium-high heat. Bring to boil, stirring constantly. Remove from heat and let cool for 10 minutes.
4. **Pour** the berry mixture over the top of the bake crust. Sprinkle top with chopped walnuts.
5. **Place** filled crust into the preheated oven and bake for 20 minutes or until berry mixture has set. Let cool and cut into squares just before serving.

* When baking with agave, honey, or molasses, lower the oven temperature by 25 degrees to avoid overbrowning.

Seasoning without salt

When you're at home, you get to season and prepare your own food. This is a huge advantage, as you know exactly what's going into your food. But it can be a bit tricky getting used for seasoning your food without salt, especially if you're used to consuming a lot of salt in a day. Food might taste a bit bland at first, but you'll get used to it, and you'll soon start to appreciate the wide variety of tastes that other herbs and spices add to your food.

First, I'm going to give a list of some seasoning products that you should cut out of your diet. Unfortunately, there are quite a few here (and a few of my personal favorites are on the list).

- Barbecue sauce
- Alfredo sauce
- Garlic, onion, and celery salt
- Mustard and ketchup
- Soy and worchestershire sauce
- Tartar sauce

There are a lot of other things that you should avoid, but these are some of the main ones. Always be sure to check the nutrition facts on the seasonings and sauces that you use! Even some low-sodium varieties can contain quite a bit of salt, so don't just trust the label.

You might be thinking that your food is going to be awfully unexciting without these seasonings, but don't worry—I'm going to recommend a few ways to replace them. First, use herbs to flavor your food; herbs are some of the healthiest things you can add to your diet, and there are actually a lot of health benefits to them that you might not be aware of. Add basil to your eggs, chili powder to your Mexican dishes, rosemary and thyme to your meats, and sage to your soups. There are a lot of spices that will add more taste, too— things like cinnamon and nutmeg in your breads, cayenne in things that need a little heat, and allspice on barbecued foods.

You can also create your own blends, which can be a lot of fun! Here are three great herb-and-spice blends from SFGate:

Basic spice

Combine paprika, black pepper, onion powder, garlic powder, thyme, sage, parsley and cayenne, and add to meat or make a paste with broth. This will add a good dash of flavor without imparting any cuisine-specific taste to your food.

Italian spice

Put a mix of basil, marjoram, garlic, oregano, rosemary, thyme, sage, savory and black pepper on any meat, or use it for your own spaghetti sauce.

Mexican spice

Chili powder, cumin, garlic powder, coriander and oregano make for a great Mexican blend that works well for meats and rice.

Of course, you can always experiment and make your own spice blend, which can be a lot of fun! When you're on the DASH diet, it's a great idea to head to the store and invest in a big batch of salt-free herbs and spices that you can use on your foods and combine to make your own blends.

Cooking with less fat

Not only does preparing your own food allow you to use less salt, but you can also make some healthy choices to reduce the amount of fat that you consume at home. Of course, the first step in this process is to buy foods that are fresh and low in fat—this will make it a lot easier. But the way in which you prepare those foods can also make a difference. Choose skinless chicken, lean cuts of other meats, and wild-caught fish, which contain healthier fats than farmed ones. Choose olive or coconut oil instead of vegetable oil when you need to.

As I mentioned before, choosing healthier methods of preparation can be very beneficial. When at all possible, choose to grill, roast, bake, or steam your foods, and avoid frying and smoking. Deep-frying is probably the worst way that you can prepare your food, so I strongly recommend avoiding that at all costs! There are some other things you can do that you might not have thought of, though. For example, using nonstick cookware can help reduce the need for butter and oil when you're cooking on the stove. Using a steamer for rice and vegetables will do the same thing. It's a small difference, but it adds up over time!

Finally, make a point to trim as much fat off of meats as you can before cooking. Even if you're going to be using one of the healthiest methods above, trimming just a bit of fat off will help keep your fat consumption down. This is especially true of saturated fats, which are often found in meats.

Conclusion

Now that you've almost finished this book, you have the knowledge that will help you embark on your own heart-healthy version of the DASH diet. Whether your goal is to reduce your blood pressure, lose weight, manage diabetes, or all three, you have the tools that will allow you to reach your goal in a healthy manner. I hope you agree that the DASH diet is one of the most sensical diets out there—I truly believe that there are no better diets on the market right now. The combination of heart-healthy, fresh foods, exercise, and an easy way of keeping track of your caloric intake is tough to beat.

The final section of this book contains a number of recipes that you can use to get started on the DASH diet. I encourage you to use these while you're getting started on the diet, as having your meal planning done for you is a huge help. Once you've become more accustomed to this style of eating, however, I recommend doing some experimenting. Try other foods, different combinations of servings, and new ways of eating. Everyone has their own requirements for how much they need to eat and when, and finding yours will be a huge help in your diet.

Finally, I'd like to encourage you to share the DASH diet with others. I mentioned in the beginning that even though the diet has received a lot of acclaim, many people still don't know about it. I strongly believe the reason for this is that the spokespeople of fad diets are a lot louder, and I think that the people who have used the DASH diet and understand its amazing simplicity and effectiveness need to speak up more. Share your results with the world, and encourage others to try out this diet. It deserves a lot more press than it gets, and I hope you'll help me give it the recognition it should be receiving!

About the Author

Patrick Dixon is a feature writer, business owner, and author with an inclination towards healthy eating. Born and raised in New Hampshire, with its lush green surroundings and landscapes that welcome exercise and peace of mind, he has always had an affinity for the outdoors and physical activities.

After suffering a heart attack many years ago, which he thankfully survived, Patrick's commitment to a healthy lifestyle intensified and has never been stronger than it is today. After that health scare, he vowed to stay fit and active, research health topics, and share his passion for health with friends, family, and the rest of the world. Remarkably, he has never strayed from this pledge.

He feels that the saying should read "The way to a man's heart health is through his stomach," because the best foods are those that keep the heart beating strong, literally.

Patrick also maintains a modest collection of musical instruments from around the world, with guitars and percussion instruments being his favorite. He now lives in California with his wife Lynn and two wonderful children, one boy and one girl. In his spare time, he enjoys cooking for his family, hiking the Hollywood hills, playing music, traveling, and unwinding with a good book.

One Last Thing...

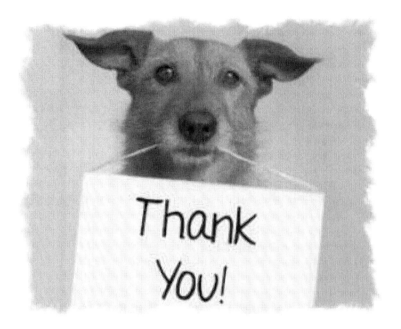

Thank you so much for reading my book. I hope you really liked it. As you probably know, many people look at the reviews before they decide to purchase a book. If you liked the book, could you please take a minute to leave a review with your feedback? 60 seconds is all I'm asking for, and it would mean the world to me.

Patrick Dixon

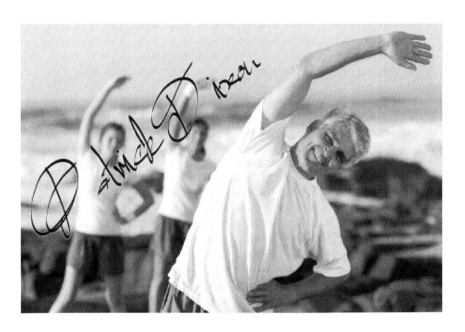

NaturalWay
Publishing

Atlanta, Georgia USA

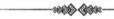